The Change of Life
Diet and Cookbook

The Change of Life Diet and Cookbook

*Delicious, Healthy Recipes to Savor Before,
During, and After Menopause*

ELAINE MAGEE, MPH, R.D.

AVERY

a member of Penguin Group (USA) Inc.

New York

Most Avery books are available at special quantity discounts for bulk purchase for sales promotions, premiums, fund-raising, and educational needs. Special books or book excerpts also can be created to fit specific needs. For details, write Penguin Group (USA) Inc. Special Markets, 375 Hudson Street, New York, NY 10014.

a member of
Penguin Group (USA) Inc.
375 Hudson Street
New York, NY 10014
www.penguin.com

Library of Congress Cataloging-in-Publication Data

Magee, Elaine.
The change of life diet and cookbook : delicious, healthy recipes to savor before,
during, and after menopause / Elaine Magee.
p.   cm.
Includes index.
ISBN 1-58333-190-5
1. Menopause—Diet therapy—Recipes.   2. Menopause—Nutritional aspects.
3. Middle-aged women—Health and hygiene.   I. Title.

RG186.M238   2004   2004043767
618.1'750654—dc22

Printed in the United States of America
1   3   5   7   9   10   8   6   4   2

This book is printed on acid-free paper. ♾

Book design by Amanda Dewey

Acknowledgments

Many thanks go to all the researchers whose study results were included in this book and who took time to answer my e-mail and phone calls. I have so much respect for the vital and tireless work that you all do. I would not have been able to offer my readers practical advice in all the various subject areas covered in this book (from diet and insomnia to food and mood to hot flash–free foods) if not for your hard work and published studies.

I would like also to thank Patricia Geraghty, N.P. (my friend, my Lamaze coach from foureen years ago, and one of the most informed and compassionate practitioners I have ever met), for her expert input on Chapters 1, 2, 5, and 9. I had a lot of fun writing Chapter 5—but Patricia's comments gave this chapter meaning.

To one of the bravest women I know—my mother.

My mother was a child in Holland during World War II; her family hid two Jewish friends under their house, and she survived many horrific ordeals during this time. In her late fifties she survived breast cancer, and she has been very active in the American Cancer Society ever since. She was selfless and unwavering in the care of my father as his health declined with every passing day. Mom, I am so proud to be your daughter—this book is for you!

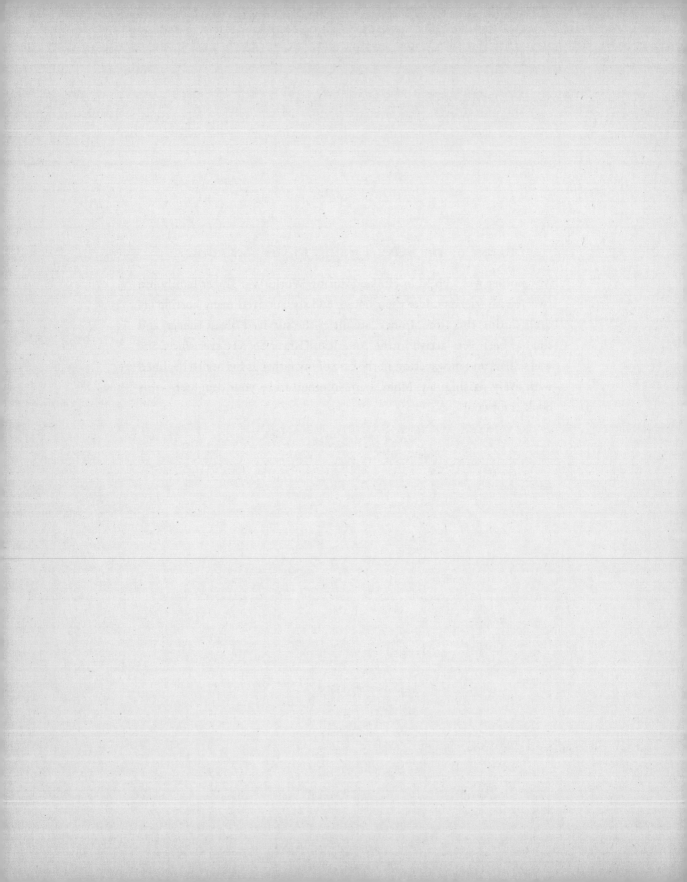

Contents

List of Recipes

The Change of Life
Diet and Cookbook

Introduction:

Feeding the Menopause Monster

The Top Seven Symptoms of Menopause—and
How to Eat Your Way Around Them!

None of us knows what perimenopause is going to be like for us personally until we are there—smack-dab in the middle of it. We can ask our mothers and aunts to get an idea based on what they experienced, but we won't know for sure until we go through our own private passage in this transitional time of our lives.

Every woman experiences different symptoms, different combinations of symptoms, and different levels of severity of symptoms during perimenopause. Some of you may be quite challenged by night sweats while others will hardly notice night symptoms. Some of you may find that your bad moods are coming more than they are going, while others are most bothered by—what was that again?—oh, yeah, your diminishing memory.

I'll Take the Breast Swelling, but the Breast Pain Has Got to Go!

You won't find a chapter of recipes on breast pain because, quite frankly, there isn't enough information on it to fill the pages. But I do want to pass along some practical tips you can try:

- Some women have increased breast pain when they are under stress, so try to set all those stress-reduction strategies in motion as soon as possible.
- Try eliminating coffee (yes, even decaffeinated) to see if this helps you—and, just so you know, hearing this hurts me just as much as it hurts you!
- Make a daily dose of flaxseed (about 1 tablespoon of ground flaxseed a day) your habit for a month and see if the breast soreness subsides. Some women find that this does the trick. And I've got to say, this certainly helps me with my breast soreness. While I was writing my flaxseed cookbook, *The Flax Cookbook,* and was testing flax recipe after flax recipe, one day I suddenly noticed my monthly— always there, like clockwork—PMS-related breast soreness had vanished.
- Some women report relief after taking a daily supplement of evening primrose oil, possibly due to the gamma-linoleic acid it contains, which has been shown to have an anti-inflammatory and analgesic effect. The dose often recommended for severe breast pain is 3 to 4 grams per day. Check with your doctor before taking any herbal or nonherbal supplements. The only trouble is, you may need to take it for three months before you feel any relief.

Whatever your symptoms, the following chapters will provide you with practical food guidance and recipes to get you started on your way to relief. Keep in mind, though, a food or lifestyle tip that works for you may not work for your friend. But here's the good news: most of the suggestions you will be reading about in the following chapters are things we should all be doing anyway in the interest of general health, like eating more nutrient-rich, higher-fiber plant foods or supplementing our smoothies with a couple teaspoons of ground flaxseed. So incorporate as many food and lifestyle tips as you can—you'll not only be more comfortable for it, you'll be healthier for it as well. And that's a good thing to be as you dance into your 50s, 60s, and 70s!

1.

Why Live HRT-Free?

Hormone replacement therapy, also known as HRT—should you take it or not? That was and continues to be the big question. There are pros and cons on each side of the HRT question, the answer to which basically comes down to each woman and her physician weighing the severity of her symptoms, her personal medical history, and her risk of certain diseases against the potential risks of HRT. The weighing of the pros and cons of HRT and the personal decision that each woman has to make hasn't changed over the years. But due to the results of The Women's Health Initiative, a large national study, we now have more information on what the real benefits are and what we truly risk by choosing to take HRT.

The Women's Health Initiative enrolled more than 16,000 women in a scientific study; half of the women took estrogen and progesterone in the form of Prempro and half of them took an inactive pill (a placebo). These women were to be observed for eight years of the study.

For women with severe and debilitating menopause symptoms, taking HRT may be unavoidable. But for most women, thankfully, menopause symptoms will be not be severe and many (hot flashes and night sweats, for instance) will be short-lived. But the long-term implications of menopause are still with us—osteoporosis and other conditions and diseases can be exacerbated by lower estrogen levels. That may leave you with a choice to make—whether or not to take HRT. If you choose to go through menopause without starting HRT, I want you to feel that you have some control over what's happening in your body and your emotions. There are many things you can do with your diet and lifestyle to discourage the most common menopause symptoms and certainly to decrease the risk of osteoporosis/bone fractures and colon cancer (the two clear benefits of taking HRT), without the use of drugs. That's what this book will help you do!

The average lifespan for women is approaching 80 years. The median age of menopause is 51 years. This means we will spend roughly 30 years (almost ⅓ of our lives) in a postmenopausal, low-estrogen state. This loss of reproductive hormones affects almost every cell in our bodies, particularly at the cardiovascular, skeletal, and reproductive levels.

Following natural menopause and the decrease of estrogen, women's bones rapidly lose strength, and the membranes of the vagina and genitalia become thinner and do not lubricate as well. We also see an increase in the number of women who develop heart disease, and risk factors for heart disease, such as increased cholesterol levels. Prior to the Women's Health Initiative study, we knew that women on estrogen and progesterone maintained stronger bones and had fewer fractures. We also knew that women on hormones postmenopausally had thicker and healthier mucous membranes in the vaginal area. Finally, women on estrogen and progesterone have lower cholesterol levels and apparently healthy vascular systems but not necessarily less heart disease.

The Women's Health Initiative was designed to confirm our existing knowledge, and to show that the lower and healthier cholesterol levels also result in less heart disease. Surprisingly, the researchers saw increased incidence of heart disease in the Prempro group over the placebo group. While the increase was not a large number of women, the study showed that we can no longer recommend estrogen and progesterone replacement therapy as a means to protect the heart. The study did confirm the benefits to both bone health and genital mucous membrane health. The Women's Health Initiative also showed a small but not statistically significant increase in the number of women who developed breast cancer in the group of women taking hormones. Other findings from the group taking hormones included an increase in blood clots, sometimes resulting in strokes, confirming that women who are at increased risk of forming blood clots should not use postmenopausal hormones. No risk of either heart disease or breast cancer was seen with short-term use of postmenopausal hormones vs. placebo.

When I wrote my first book on menopause, *Eat Well for a Healthy Menopause,* in 1996, I pointed out the potential side effects and health risks of HRT. After writing the book, I remember deciding that I, personally, would try my best to manage menopause without hormones when the time came. My decision was carefully thought through. My mother was one of the many women in her generation to automatically go on hormone replacement therapy at the first sign of menopause. Years later, she was diagnosed with nongenetic breast cancer at the age of 58 and was immediately taken off HRT. She had breast surgery followed by six months of chemotherapy. That was twelve years ago.

In 2000, U.S. pharmacists filled 22 million prescriptions for Prempro, an HRT regimen that includes estrogen plus progestin. That's a whole lot of hormone replacement therapy! But all this has changed. Due to the results from The Women's Health Initiative study, federal health officials felt strongly enough about the increased risks to cardiovascular health due to this therapy that they announced that Prempro does significantly more harm than good when taken for long periods. After five years of study on more than 27,000 women, researchers found conclusively that the combination of hormones in Prempro *raises* the risk of heart attack, stroke, blood clots, and breast cancer.

Hello! Stop the bus! What did they just say? HRT is more harmful to our heart than helpful? In fact, the researchers actually cut the study short (it was supposed to run eight years), because the results were so decisive and disturbing. After just one year, researchers started seeing possible risks along with benefits. But, as the study went on, the ratio of risks to benefits grew worse and worse.

Although Prempro was the form of estrogen and progesterone used in The Women's Health Initiative study, another large study published in Britain in August 2003, the Million Women Study, measured the effects of many forms of estrogen and progesterone on the risk of breast cancer. They found a small increase in the cases of breast cancer in the hormone group, similar to the number seen in the Women's Health Initiative, regardless of the type of estrogen or progesterone used by the women in the study. The form of estrogen and progesterone used does not alter the risk. No increased risk of breast cancer was seen, though, with short-term use of hormones compared to a placebo.

You Do the Math

As the lists below show, the risks of HRT do appear to outweigh the benefits.

HRT Benefits
+ The women taking HRT had ⅓ fewer incidence of hip fracture compared to the women in the placebo control group.
+ The women who took HRT suffered significantly fewer incidences of colon cancer than those in the placebo control group.

HRT Risks
- The heart attack rate was 29 percent higher in the HRT group compared to the control group.
- Risk of pulmonary blood clots were higher throughout the study in the HRT group compared to the control group.
- Stroke risk was high from the second year on (the stroke rate was 41 percent higher in the HRT group compared to those not taking hormone therapy).
- Five years into the study, it became clear that women on Prempro were developing invasive breast cancer at a higher rate (26 percent higher) than the control group.

More Sobering Facts About HRT

There are two general indications for HRT use: treatment of some menopausal symptoms and the prevention of osteoporosis.

The Bones: Risks vs. Benefits

After two to three years of hormone therapy, clinical trials show 5 to 7 percent greater spinal bone density in women randomly selected to take HRT compared to those randomly assigned to take a placebo.

However, in one of the largest trials with fracture outcomes, the HERS (Heart and Estrogen/Progestin Replacement) study, hormone therapy appeared to be most effective in reducing fracture risk in women who already had abnormal bone density (osteoporosis) at the beginning of the trial than in women with normal bone density ("Effect of alendronate on risk of fracture in women with low bone density but without vertebral fractures"). One of the other take home messages from the HERS study was that another medication for osteoporosis, alendronate, was more effective for people with existing osteoporosis than postmenopausal hormones. Alendronate is taken by mouth for prevention or treatment of osteoporosis. It slows the rate of bone breakdown and increases bone thickness in the small bones of the spine and hip. There are many other medications available to women today for treating and slowing down osteoporosis that have nothing to do with HRT. You can discuss your options with your practitioner.

The Health Costs

One of the health costs of HRT is an increased risk of heart disease events, such as heart attack and stroke, if you already have heart disease. HERS (Heart and Estrogen/Progestin Replacement Study), a randomized, blinded (the participants don't know which group they are in), placebo-controlled trial among 2,763 postmenopausal women with documented Coronary Heart Disease (CHD) in 1998, found no overall benefit of four years of treatment with estrogen plus progestin, and women in the HRT group had a 50 percent increase in risk of coronary heart disease (CHD) events during the first year of therapy.

Another study, the Estrogen Replacement in Atherosclerosis study, found that neither unopposed estrogen (estrogen taken without progestin) nor estrogen plus progestin slowed the progression of atherosclerosis (accumulation of lipids and other substances in the artery walls) measured by quantitative angiography among 309 women with preexisting coronary heart disease. An angiogram is a common procedure performed to evaluate the heart. It allows doctors to see whether the arteries are blocked. A local anesthetic is injected into the groin and then very thin tubing is inserted into an artery. The tubing is pushed upward until it enters blood vessels in the heart.

It has also been found that there is an increased risk of heart disease in women *without* preexisting coronary heart disease. The Women's Health Initiative HRT study, 2002, the randomized trial we mentioned earlier, which studied more than 27,000 women (98 percent of whom did not have preexisting coronary heart disease at the start of the trial), recently reported that both unopposed estrogen and estrogen plus progestin were associated with an increased risk of cardiovascular events compared to placebo during the first three years of treatment.

There is also an increased risk of stroke for people taking HRT. The Women's Estrogen for Stroke Trial, 2001, also found no reduction in risk of stroke and death or coronary events among 664 postmenopausal women treated with estradiol (a form of estrogen) or placebo for 2.8 years. In fact, the researchers found that the incidence of death due to stroke was higher in the estrogen group and that the nonfatal strokes in that group were associated with slightly worse neurological and functional impairments at one month after stroke. The risk of stroke within the first six months after enrollment in the study was also higher among women in the estrogen group.

There is also an increased risk of breast cancer for those who take HRT. Hormone use for more than five years is associated with a 30 to 60 percent increase in risk of breast cancer.

Estrogen promotes tumor induction and growth in animals and increases the growth rate of human breast cells in vitro (test tubes).

There is an increased risk of venous thromboembolism. (A *thrombus* is a clot that can develop in a vein. If the clot detaches and circulates in the blood vessels, it is called an *embolus*. The embolus is dangerous and potentially deadly if it gets caught and fills or blocks a blood vessel in the heart, lungs, or brain.) Hormone therapy has been shown to increase the risk of venous thromboembolism by three times the rate of women who are not taking hormone therapy.

And HRT is also associated with an increased risk of gallbladder disease. Hormone therapy has been shown to increase the risk of gallbladder disease by about 40 percent of the rate of women not taking hormone therapy.

What HRT Doesn't Do

No randomized trial of hormone therapy has shown it to reduce the risk of coronary events, such as chest pain and heart attack, in any group of postmenopausal women. This lack of evidence recently led the American Heart Association to revise their guidelines to recommend against initiating use of HRT for secondary prevention of cardiovascular disease, a reversal of their position taken when HRT first came into use.

In addition, postmenopausal hormone therapy should not be used for treatment of major depression, but it might improve depressive symptoms indirectly by relieving hot flashes and improving sleep. And hormone therapy has not been shown to be effective for some other symptoms of menopause, such as unstable moods, memory loss, and decreased libido.

The above findings and studies have given millions of women pause, including myself. After reading this list and weighing my own personal health history, I have chosen to forfeit the possible health benefits of HRT and instead make the changes in my diet and lifestyle to decrease bone fracture risk and reduce my risk of colon cancer (including a colonoscopy every ten years starting at age 50), rather than take HRT and increase my risk of heart attack, pulmonary blood clots, strokes, and possibly breast cancer.

In *The Change of Life Diet and Cookbook,* you will discover powerful recipes and nutrition suggestions to decrease your risk of bone fracture (Chapter 9) and colon cancer (Chapter 10) through diet and lifestyle changes instead of relying on HRT. But what about the myriad menacing menopausal symptoms—night sweats, depression, hot flashes—that cause most women to turn to HRT in the first place? The majority of the recipe chapters in *The Change of Life Diet and Cookbook* are designed specifically to tackle the eight most common menopausal symptoms.

What About the Recipes?

The Change of Life Diet and Cookbook does three vital things differently from many of the menopause cookbooks you may have already seen.

1. The recipes are arranged by menopause symptoms and disease-prevention benefits so you can easily find the information you need when you need it. Most menopause-based cookbooks arrange recipes by food categories.
2. This book features practical, easy-to-make recipes that allow you to follow my food suggestions while also enjoying your favorite foods. Some menopause cookbooks include labor-intensive recipes for dishes that most of us wouldn't recognize or be interested in eating or making.
3. All recipes include the basic nutrition information (calories; grams of protein, carbohydrate, and fat; the breakdown of saturated fat, monounsaturated fat, and polyunsaturated fat, as well as milligrams of cholesterol; the percent of calories from fat; sodium content; and grams of fiber) along with the amount of omega-3 and omega-6 fatty acids; amounts of antioxidants; and milligrams of calcium and iron. The majority of the menopause cookbooks already on the market do *not* include nutritional analysis with the recipes, a critical piece of information.

This book contains real recipes for real women—women who have busy lives, happily filled with careers and hobbies, women who enjoy vegetarian dishes sometimes but also like to have their beef and eat it too, women who crave comfort foods more often than not, women who tend to shop at the big chain grocery store down the street, and women who have a microwave and aren't afraid to use it. Let's eat and be HRT-free!

2.

Is It Me, or Is It Hot in Here?

Eating to Ease Hot Flashes

If you've turned to this chapter, chances are pretty good you are one of the eight out of ten women who will experience hot flashes during perimenopause. Hot flashes are the most common uncomfortable symptom of perimenopause.

A hot flash is caused by a physiological series of events and changes. During perimenopause, estrogen levels change, (usually a sudden decrease), resulting in a change in the body's circulation. A hot flash starts in the area of the brain that regulates body temperature. Your face and/or upper body suddenly feel warm, leading to blushing and sometimes rapid and profuse sweating. Then your heart beats faster. By the end of the hot flash, you may feel a cold chill as the sweat evaporates.

Find the Pattern, and You Can Start Planning Ahead!

A hot flash can last from one minute to five or ten minutes. You can even be hit with a flurry of hot flashes a few minutes apart. Sounds similar to labor contractions, doesn't it?

Hot flashes usually have a consistent pattern, hitting you hard at a certain time of day. Each woman's pattern is unique. Some find that the afternoon is their peak time for hot flashes, while others have trouble early in the morning or late at night. It may be helpful to write down the times you have hot flashes. If you do notice a pattern, use it to your advantage! When you know your pattern, you can plan ahead to discourage hot flashes at this particular time as much as possible. Some ways to head off a hot flash include:

- Dress in layers. Take off your outer layer of clothing ahead of time to keep your body temperature as cool as is comfortably possible. A small fan at work might be a good idea, too.
- Sip cool beverages at times when your hot flashes might start to keep your body's core temperature cooler in advance.
- Stop drinking hot beverages around this time.
- Avoid spicy foods around your prime hot-flash time. Follow the Hot Flash Food Hints below as much as possible.
- Eat smaller-sized meals! Large meals can increase your body temperature. When you eat a large meal, particularly one that is also high in fat, your body's digestive system has to work extra hard digesting and metabolizing, all of which generates extra heat.
- Chew on some ice chips. Keep a glass of ice chips on your desk at work or next to your bed at night. At your most vulnerable hot-flash times, chew on some ice periodically to keep your body temperature down as much as possible.
- Take a cold shower. Some women find that if they take a long, cold shower or twenty-minute cool bath first thing in the morning or right before bed at night, it keeps them almost hot flash–free for hours afterward.
- Reduce the stress in your life. I know that's easier said than done. You might be thinking the only stress you have is your hot flashes, but high stress can be a hot-flash trigger for some.

Hot Flash Food Hints

Can what you eat and drink encourage or discourage hot flashes? The short answer is *yes,* although as usual, different things help different people. Some women swear that eating or drinking one to two servings of soy a day keeps hot flashes at bay, and others have had success with one to two tablespoons of ground flaxseed a day.

The good news is that these foods may help decrease the frequency and the severity of hot flashes; the bad news is that they may not make them disappear entirely. Eating soy and other isoflavone-rich foods also may help women with milder symptoms more than women with more severe symptoms.

Since my personal plan of attack for perimenopause is to avoid HRT at all costs, I plan to cover my nutritional and lifestyle bases by incorporating as many of the following suggestions into my life as practically possible to find what helps my specific hot-flash situation. All the food hints below are healthy things to do for your body with or without hot flashes, so why not do them no matter what?

I've grouped some of these helpful Hot Flash Food Hints into two categories: foods to choose and foods to lose. Sometimes it isn't what you add to your diet but what you take away that helps!

Foods to Choose

- A daily serving or two of phytoestrogen-rich soy, such as soymilk, tofu, miso, soynuts, and edamame.
- Other phytoestrogen-rich foods, such as papaya, peas, beans, and lentils.
- Ground flaxseed. Flaxseed pumps quite a few powerful substances into our diet—fiber, plant-derived omega-3s, and phytochemicals. But in the case of hot flashes, the fact that flaxseed is the richest food source on the planet of the phytoestrogen lignan is what really puts it on the map. Generally one tablespoon of ground flaxseed a day, considered safe and effective by experts, seems to be very helpful to women. Ground flaxseed is best kept in the freezer, so if you buy whole flaxseeds, grind a month's supply, then keep it in a bag or container in the freezer. Just take out what you need every day.

Foods to Lose

Some women find some relief from hot flashes by avoiding certain foods and beverages, and some of these items are going to be painful to give up. That morning cup of java, for example, may be triggering some of your hot flashes. And that's not all—there are several other favorite foods that could be hot-flash triggers.

The big three trigger foods are:

- hot and spicy foods
- foods with caffeine
- alcohol

Note: You may also find that hot drinks and possibly hot soups seem to trigger hot flashes.

Avoid these foods at certain times of the day, or all day if necessary. When you have a hot flash or series of hot flashes, consider whether you had one of the trigger foods minutes before or a few hours before. Hot and spicy foods and hot drinks tend to have an almost immediate effect on hot flashes, while alcohol and caffeine can affect you thirty minutes or even two to four hours later.

Soy Is Good for You

We keep hearing about the power of the bean called soy. The American Heart Association recently stated that 25 to 50 grams of soy a day can help lower LDL ("bad") cholesterol by as much as 8 percent. Other studies have shown promising results for soy's benefits in reducing risk of stroke, cancer, osteoporosis, and hot flashes. One recent study reported that eating a diet rich in soy products may cut the risk of breast cancer in half.

Note: If you think you may have any of these conditions, see your doctor before making any big changes to your diet.

What gives soy its nutritional power? There is some debate among researchers over whether it is the isoflavonoids/isoflavones (phytoestrogens) in soy that give it all these health benefits or if it is the soy protein and fat—or all three. Either way, the bottom line is that you should eat one or two servings of soy per day. Several times a week may be a good start for people who normally don't have soy at all.

Mark Messina, Ph.D., M.S., a well-known author and lecturer on soy, recommends a daily serving of soy (i.e., one cup of soymilk or four ounces of tofu) to people in general. For every gram of soy protein you get from a traditional soy food (such as tofu, soymilk, miso, tempeh, soybeans, and soynuts), you also get about 3½ mg of isoflavones. So a serving of soymilk or tofu (about 8–10 grams of soy protein) will give you roughly 28–35 mg of isoflavones.

How Does Soy Work on Hot Flashes?

There is much to understand about soy and hot flashes. In fact, the jury is still out on soy. But several studies do suggest that soy and soy products may help relieve mild, uncomfortable hot-flash episodes. The plant estrogens in soy may help stabilize the changes in estrogen levels that can lead to hot flashes.

Isoflavones are phytoestrogens (plant estrogens) that have a chemical structure similar to regular estrogen, so the phytoestrogens appear to latch on to some of the estrogen receptors in the body. But they don't turn these receptors on (by opening up the actions of estrogen) to the same degree as regular estrogen. And that's only the beginning. Once the phytoestrogens bind (like a key in a lock) to these receptors and act as estrogen in the body but not as consistently as a woman's own estrogen, they keep regular estrogen from binding to it—which can have various desirable health effects. The two most active isoflavones are genistein and daidzein. Basically, these phytoestrogens have some of the same positive effects as human estrogen without some of its negative effects. Some studies suggest that these isoflavones can help dampen hot flashes and may be one of the factors (along with fiber) that contribute to soy's ability to help reduce cardiovascular risk.

CAN ISOFLAVONES LOWER BREAST CANCER RISK?

A recent study reported that the women with the most isoflavones in their diet had the lowest risk of breast cancer—and this was especially true of postmenopausal women.

The Whole Foods, and Nothing but the Whole Foods

There have been a few disappointing studies on the perimenopausal benefits of soy but, depending on who you talk to, the overwhelming data is in soy's favor. Some studies suggest it's the whole food that's most effective, not the isoflavones alone. There may be a special synergy between the various soy components. (And the same may be true for other phytoestrogen-rich foods.) One Wake Forest University study compared the effect of isoflavone supplements vs. soy foods in reducing hot flashes—and soy foods won! I suspect it's the whole package of benefits that makes soy most impressive for peri- and post-menopause.

Well, there has never been a better time to try and work some soy into your daily diet. Soy has come a long way, baby! It's not just in health-food stores anymore, and it isn't just tofu, either. There are many ways you can easily and conveniently get a serving of soy from your local supermarket. Tofu now comes in firm, soft, and silken varieties, and is available baked in marinades of various flavors or smoked. Then there is soymilk, which is not only available in several brands now, but also comes in various flavors like vanilla and chocolate. And I haven't even started talking about the frozen food section—there are several soy offerings there! And more and more snacks and cereals are available fortified with soy.

But, remember, to get the most from soy, eat whole soy foods not soy supplements. They give you fiber and other important nutrients along with isoflavones. And it may be that the beneficial effects of soy have to do not with one component of soy but with the combination of substances in soy.

The term "soy" includes all products that originate from the soybean. Here they are; I've included my opinion of each of them.

The Top Eight Ways to Get Some Soy

1. **Green soybeans**, sometimes called edamame, are available in the frozen vegetable section shelled or in pods.

ELAINE'S TAKE:
I love this soy option. They look like baby lima beans and have a mild taste and a nice texture that is firmer than canned beans.

How Can I Add Them to Recipes?

- Use cooked, shelled green soybeans in recipes in place of beans such as in soups and casseroles.
- You can lightly microwave the pods. (Cook about 2 cups of pods on high in the microwave with ¼ cup of water in a covered dish until tender, about 5–7 minutes.) Chill and then eat as an appetizer or snack, discarding the pods and eating the green soybeans inside.
- You can lightly micro-cook the shelled soybeans, sprinkle with some salt and pepper and a tiny bit of butter or canola margarine, and eat warm.

2. **Canned soybeans** can be found in some supermarkets.

Elaine's Take:
I haven't been impressed with the brands that I've tasted. But maybe there is a better tasting brand out there that I haven't tried or one that suits your taste.

How Can I Add Them to Recipes?

- Use canned soybeans in recipes where you would use other canned beans, such as in bean salads, bean soups, and entrées made with beans.

3. **Tofu** can be found in the refrigerated section either in the produce section or near the dairy area. There are many types available: firm, soft, light, or silken.

Elaine's Take:
I personally like tofu. There are two ways to approach tofu: the hide-it technique, where you hope that no one will notice it's in there, or featuring it as one of the premier ingredients in your dish. I do both on a regular basis.

How Can I Add It to Recipes?

- You can add it to stir-fry dishes or casseroles or other main entrées in place of some or all of the meat ingredients. If you buy the soft or silken tofu, you can add it to sauces, soups, smoothies, dips, or spreads.

4. **Baked tofu** can often be found where fresh tofu is sold and is available in several different flavors, such spicy or sesame.

Elaine's Take:

I especially like the baked tofu, because it is so convenient—it's flavored and can be eaten immediately or added to recipes without any preparation or seasonings and sauces.

How Can I Add It to Recipes?

- You can literally eat this just as it is, with crackers, or you can add it to a sandwich spread, to the filling of a vegetarian burrito, or to any other mixed dish or casserole.

5. **Soymilk (plain or flavored)** can often be found in the dairy section of your supermarket. There are several national brands available, and each brand usually offers plain, vanilla, and chocolate soymilk.

Elaine's Take:

Some soymilks taste better than others. I have found a couple brands that work for me; Silk brand is my favorite.

How Can I Add It to Recipes?

- You can add soymilk to cold cereal, make your hot oatmeal with it, or add it to iced or hot coffee, shakes, and smoothies. If you are using it to make instant pudding, use half soymilk and half cow's milk; otherwise the pudding may not thicken as well. You can also drink the chocolate or vanilla soymilk as a beverage once a day.

6. **Soy flour** can be found in the flour/baking section of some supermarkets and in most health-food stores.

Elaine's Take:

I was surprised that soy flour wasn't bad at all in place of some of the flour in various bread or muffin recipes. I tried it in all sorts of recipes, and sometimes people could notice the difference and sometimes they couldn't. But for the most part, everyone still seemed to enjoy the foods I made with it. It adds a light yellow color, a slightly heavier texture, and a somewhat "yeasty" flavor.

How Can I Add It to Recipes?

- For each cup of flour, you can replace 3 to 4 tablespoons of the flour with soy flour. This means if a recipe calls for 2 cups of flour, you can add about ⅓ to ½ cup of soy flour and 1½ to 1⅔ cups of white flour.

7. **Soynuts** can be found in the health-food, bulk, snacks, or produce section of your supermarket and in most health-food stores.

Elaine's Take:

Not only do I like crunching on these nuts when I need a little snack, but I find myself adding them to all sorts of dishes—from salads to trail mix. They come in several flavors, such as apple cinnamon, BBQ, plain, and more.

How Can I Add Them to Recipes?

- I tend to add the plain flavored toasted soynuts to recipes so that I'm not overloading the recipe with the strong seasonings from the flavored soynuts. In many recipes you can sprinkle them on top as a crunchy topping and (depending on the particular recipe) you can add them in place of nuts or seeds.

8. **Soy dairylike products** can be found in the alternative dairy section in many supermarkets; in my supermarket they are in the regular dairy section. Depending on where you live, you might find a soy alternative to cream cheese, sour cream, cheese, ice cream, and yogurt.

Elaine's Take:

The soy cream cheese I tried had a slight yellowish tint to it, which might be unappealing to those of you who usually eat very white cream cheese. I very much enjoyed the Scallion-Soy Cream Cheese (recipe on page 145) that I blended together. So far I have liked all the dishes I have used the soy cream cheese in.

How Can I Add It to Recipes?

- Depending on the recipe, you can add soy cream cheese in place of all or part of the regular cream cheese you would normally add—in spreads and dips, cream cheese glaze for cinnamon rolls, filling for stuffed chicken, etc. You may not want to use it in your cheesecake, though; a small tub of soy cream cheese is quite expensive, and most cheesecake recipes call for 24 ounces of cream cheese. Plus, the soy cream cheese may not perform as well as light cream cheese in the blending and the baking.

Four Other Ways to Work in Soy

1. Order **miso soup** in Japanese restaurants or buy some in Asian specialty markets or health-food stores and heat it up at home.
2. Try **tempeh** (made from fermented soybeans). I had a difficult time finding tempeh where I live, but it tends to be available in specialty markets and health-food stores. You can use it in recipes as you would tofu.
3. **Soy burgers and meat-alternative products,** such as veggie meatballs, lunchmeat, and hot dogs, tend to use soy protein in their formulations. Check the label for some of these products to know if the one you are looking at contains soy. Some of these meat-alternative products taste better than others. Ask around to find out which of these products you should try first.
4. **Soy protein powder** can be added to smoothies, shakes, breakfast drinks, cream-based soups, and anything else that strikes your fancy.

Beyond Soy

Soy isn't the only isoflavone game in town. Isoflavones can be found in various fruits, vegetables, beans, and whole grains. Lignans are another group of phytoestrogens that may help hot flashes. Ground flaxseed is by far the richest plant source of lignans on the planet; you'll find them in assorted fruits, vegetables, and whole grains, too.

The Beneficial Bean

Beans in general are good sources of isoflavones. People don't know that, because soy seems to have gotten much of the good publicity lately, but yellow split peas, black beans, baby limas, anasazi beans, red kidney beans, red lentils, black-eyed peas, pinto beans, mung beans, adzuki beans, fava beans, and great northern beans also contain those desirable phytoestrogens, along with the phytoestrogen lignans.

Phytoestrogen-rich Fruits

The following fruits contain isoflavonoids (I) and/or lignans (L).

Apples (I)	Grapes (I)
Berries (i.e., raspberries and blackberries) (I)	Pears (L)
	Plums
Citrus fruits (I)	Strawberries (I)

Phytoestrogen-rich Vegetables

The following vegetables contain isoflavonoids (I) and/or lignans (L).

Asparagus (L)	Leeks (L)
Beets (L)	Lettuce, all types except iceberg (I)
Bell Peppers (I, L)	Iceberg lettuce (L)
Broccoli (I, L)	Onions (L)
Cabbage (I)	Snow Peas (L)
Carrots (I, L)	Squash (I, L)
Cauliflower (L)	Sweet Potatoes (L)
Cucumbers (I)	Tomatoes (I)
Eggplant (I)	Turnips (L)
Garlic (I, L)	Yams (I)

Recipes Not to Flush By

You are probably guessing that you are going to find some tofu recipes in this chapter. You are right! But I'm also giving you some recipes that will introduce soy flour to you (try it, you'll like it), along with soynuts, soymilk, green soybeans (edamame), and some high-phytoestrogen vegetables. I wanted to give you a variety of recipes that incorporate the helpful Hot Flash Food Hints we discussed above. So dive right in!

Breakfast Burrito

Makes 2 burritos • Serving size: 1 burrito

1 teaspoon canola oil

¼ cup chopped onion

½ cup chopped bell pepper

½ cup soft tofu, crumbled (firm tofu can be substituted)

½ cup egg substitute (or use 1 large egg beaten with 2 egg whites, if desired)

3 ounces turkey breakfast sausage or 97% Light Jimmy Dean Sausage, crumbled up and cooked over medium heat until nicely browned and cooked throughout, (or)

3 strips turkey bacon, cooked until crisp and broken into small bits

⅛ cup bottled or fresh salsa (mild or hot, depending on your preference)

¼ cup reduced-fat cheddar cheese

2 9-inch flour tortillas (approximately 68 grams with 160 calories and 0.5 grams fat each)

GARNISH (OPTIONAL):

½ avocado, thinly sliced

¼ cup bottled or fresh salsa

¼ cup fat-free or light sour cream

1. Add canola oil to medium nonstick frying pan over medium heat. Sauté onions, bell pepper, and tofu for about 3 minutes, stirring often.
2. Pour in the egg substitute and continue to cook, stirring frequently, until eggs are cooked throughout (1–2 minutes). Turn off heat and stir in the cooked sausage or bacon, salsa, and cheese. Cover pan and let sit 1–2 minutes.
3. Meanwhile, soften the tortillas by warming them in the microwave on high for 1 minute or in a large nonstick frying pan over medium heat.
4. Spoon half the egg mixture into the center of one of the flour tortillas and roll up like a burrito. Repeat with remaining tortilla. Garnish each serving with sliced avocado, and a dollop of salsa and sour cream if desired.

Nutritional Facts *(per serving):* 332 calories, 23 g protein, 30 g carbohydrate, 14 g fat (4.5 g saturated fat, 4.2 g monounsaturated fat, 2.6 g polyunsaturated fat, 0.3 g omega-3 fatty acids, 2.3 g omega-6 fatty acids), 44 mg cholesterol, 3 g fiber, 880 mg sodium. Calories from fat: 38 percent.

123 RE vitamin A, 38 mg vitamin C, 21 IU vitamin D, 3 IU vitamin E, 1.4 mcg vitamin B$_{12}$, 52 mcg folate, 204 mg calcium, 0.8 mcg selenium.

Hot Flash Frittata with Asparagus and Red Peppers

I like the idea of eating the frittata cold on hot days! The bright green asparagus and yellow or red bell peppers make for a beautifully colorful frittata. You get two different phytoestrogens from the aparagus, bell peppers, and garlic in this recipe. *Makes 6 large servings*

2 pounds thin asparagus, trimmed and cut diagonally into ¼-inch-wide slices

2 large yellow or red bell peppers, cut into ¼-inch-wide slices

3 shallots, minced

3 scallions, thinly sliced

1 tablespoon canola or olive oil

1 tablespoon garlic, minced

5 eggs (use higher-omega-3 eggs if available in your supermarket)

1¼ cups egg substitute

½ cup soymilk (or lowfat or whole milk, or fat-free half-and-half)

1 tablespoon Wondra quick-mixing flour

3 tablespoons chopped fresh flat-leaf parsley

1 teaspoon salt

¼ teaspoon freshly ground black pepper

1. Preheat oven to 350 degrees. Coat a 13x9x2-inch glass baking dish with canola oil cooking spray.

2. Have a bowl of ice water ready. In a large saucepan, blanch asparagus in boiling salted water for about 1 minute. Drain in colander and immediately transfer to ice water for two minutes to stop cooking. Drain asparagus well in colander and pat dry. (You can microwave the asparagus for about 2 minutes instead, if you like.)

3. In a large nonstick skillet or frying pan, cook bell peppers and shallots in 1 tablespoon of olive oil over moderately low heat, stirring occasionally, until the peppers are softened (about 5–8 minutes). About halfway through, stir in the minced garlic.

4. In a large mixing bowl, beat together the 5 eggs and 1¼ cup egg substitute. Blend 2 tablespoons of the soymilk with the flour to make a paste. Stir in the remaining milk. Add the milk mixture, along with the parsley, salt, and pepper, to the eggs and beat until blended.

5. Stir in the asparagus, bell pepper mixture, and pour into the prepared dish. Bake in the middle of the oven until golden and set (about 35 minutes). Cool frittata on a rack.

This can be served warm, or cooled in the refrigerator. (You can make the frittata a day ahead of time and cover it when chilling in the refrigerator.)

Nutritional Facts *(per serving)*: 175 calories, 15 g protein, 14 g carbohydrate, 7 g fat (1.5 g saturated fat, 0.3 g monounsaturated fat, 1.5 g polyunsaturated fat, 0.3 g omega-3 fatty acids, 1.2 g omega-6 fatty acids), 177 mg cholesterol, 4 g fiber, 550 mg sodium. Calories from fat: 36 percent.

465 RE vitamin A, 98 mg vitamin C, 45 IU vitamin D, 7.3 IU vitamin E, 1.2 mcg vitamin B_{12}, 259 mcg folate, 107 mg calcium, 0.17 mcg selenium.

Lemon–Poppy Seed Waffles

I happen to be the proud owner of a Meyer lemon tree that each year reaches its peak harvest in the middle of winter. So in January, I find myself with a big bowl of lemons just waiting to be zested. These are a complete and total hit from dad to youngest daughter.

Makes about 12 waffle squares (about 6 servings) • Serving size: 2 square waffles

1⅛ cups unbleached flour
⅓ cup soy flour
½ cup powdered sugar
2 tablespoons poppy seeds
2 teaspoons baking powder
1 teaspoon baking soda
¼ teaspoon salt
2 eggs

¼ cup egg substitute or 2 egg whites
1¼ cups plus 2 tablespoons lowfat
    buttermilk
2 tablespoons canola oil
4 teaspoons grated lemon zest (zest from
    about 2 lemons)
Fresh fruit or other assorted toppings
    (optional)

1. Add flours, sugar, poppy seeds, baking powder, baking soda, and salt to mixing bowl and beat on low to blend.
2. Add eggs, buttermilk, canola oil, and lemon zest to mixing bowl and beat on low until just blended together.
3. Let mixture stand 15 minutes (this is important because it gives the baking powder and baking soda a chance to interact with the buttermilk to produce some bubbles in the batter).

4. Preheat waffle iron according to manufacturer's instructions. When ready, lightly spray iron with canola oil cooking spray. Spoon batter onto waffle iron (use the amount recommended by the manufacturer. For my waffle iron it is ⅓ cup per square). Cover and cook until golden and cooked through. Cooking time will vary, depending on your waffle iron.

5. Repeat with remaining batter. Serve immediately with fresh fruit and/or assorted toppings!

Nutritional Facts *(per serving)*: 256 calories, 10 g protein, 33.5 g carbohydrate, 9 g fat (1.5 g saturated fat, 3.7 g monounsaturated fat, 2.6 g polyunsaturated fat, 0.5 g omega-3 fatty acids, 2.1 g omega-6 fatty acids), 74 mg cholesterol, 2 g fiber, 540 mg sodium. Calories from fat: 32 percent.

42 RE vitamin A, 2 mg vitamin C, 11 IU vitamin D, 2.1 IU vitamin E, 0.4 mcg vitamin B_{12}, 51 mcg folate, 206 mg calcium, 13 mcg selenium.

Strawberries-and-Cream Oatmeal

This recipe calls for a microwave, but the oatmeal can be cooked over medium heat in a small nonstick saucepan on the stove.   *Makes 1 serving size: about 1¼ cup*

⅓ *cup quick oats (I use Sun Country brand)*
⅔ *cup vanilla soymilk (I use Silk brand)*
dash of salt

½ *cup chopped fresh or frozen strawberries (or ¼ cup chopped dried strawberries— these are available now in some supermarkets)*
sprinkling of granulated sugar (optional)

1. Combine oats, soymilk, salt, and strawberries in a 2-cup microwave-safe bowl and stir well.

2. Microwave on high for 2 minutes. Stir, then microwave another 2 minutes if not thickened yet. Stir and microwave another minute until thickened if necessary. Mix well before serving.

Nutritional Facts (*per serving*): 199 calories, 9 g protein, 31 g carbohydrate, 4.5 g fat (1.3 g saturated fat, 0.6 g monounsaturated fat, 0.7 g polyunsaturated fat, 0.1 g omega-3 fatty acids, 0.1 g omega-6 fatty acids), 0 mg cholesterol, 5 grams fiber, 65 mg sodium. Calories from fat: 20 percent.

75 RE vitamin A, 58 mg vitamin C, 80 IU vitamin D, 0.6 IU vitamin E, 2 mcg vitamin B_{12}, 42 mcg folate, 229 mg calcium, 0.7 mcg selenium.

Soynut Snack Mix

This is a lower fat version of the Chex snack mix recipe, with some soynuts thrown in. This recipe requires a microwave.

Makes 9 cups • Serving size: 1 cup

3½ cups Crispix cereal	*1½ tablespoons maple syrup*
3½ cups Wheat Chex cereal	*¼ teaspoon garlic powder*
1 cup soynuts (plain, unflavored)	*¼ teaspoon onion powder*
2 cups mini-twist pretzels	*2 teaspoons lemon juice*
1½ tablespoons margarine, melted	*4 teaspoons Worcestershire sauce*

1. Combine cereals, soynuts, and pretzels in a large microwave-safe bowl.
2. Stir together margarine, maple syrup, garlic powder, onion powder, lemon juice, and Worcestershire sauce in a 2-cup measuring cup. Gently drizzle over cereal mixture and stir until cereal is well coated.
3. Microwave on high for 4 minutes (you may need to microwave longer, depending on your microwave), stirring after 2 minutes. Spread on paper towels to cool. Store in airtight container.

Nutritional Facts (*per cup*): 208 calories, 9 g protein, 36 g carbohydrate, 4 g fat (0.8 g saturated fat, 1 g monounsaturated fat, 0.7 g polyunsaturated fat, 0.4 g omega-3 fatty acids, 0.1 g omega-6 fatty acids), 0 mg cholesterol, 4.2 g fiber, 429 mg sodium. Calories from fat: 17 percent.

105 RE vitamin A, 8 mg vitamin C, 16 IU vitamin D, 0.3 IU vitamin E, 0.4 mcg vitamin B_{12}, 127 mcg folate, 60 mg calcium, 2 mcg selenium.

Cabbage and Sesame Tofu Salad with Crunchy Topping

This recipe originally called for ⅓ cup of butter, sesame seeds, and almonds before it is baked until crispy in the oven. I cut this down to 1 tablespoon and heated it with a few tablespoons of apple juice and half of the ramen soup powder to make a very flavorful mixture to coat the crunchies with. This works wonderfully. In fact, I've got to warn you, don't start sampling the crispies when they come out of the oven or you are likely to have very little left for the salad, as they are addictive! It takes about 22 minutes to bake the crunchy topping.

Makes 6 large servings

1 head Napa cabbage, finely shredded
    (about 12 cups)

2 cups sesame tofu (baked sesame-flavor
    tofu), diced

1 bunch green onions (white and part
    of green), thinly sliced

1 tablespoon butter

3 tablespoons apple juice

½ packet of ramen soup broth powder

1 (3-ounce) package ramen noodles
    (any flavor), broken

2 tablespoons sesame seeds

½ cup slivered almonds

DRESSING:

3 tablespoons cider vinegar

2 tablespoons canola oil

4 tablespoons light corn syrup

2 tablespoons light soy sauce

½ packet ramen soup broth powder

1. Combine cabbage with tofu and green onions in very large bowl. Cover and refrigerate until ready to serve.

2. Preheat oven to 350 degrees and line a baking sheet or jelly roll pan with foil. Coat the foil with canola oil cooking spray.

3. Melt butter and mix with apple juice and ½ packet of ramen broth powder in small nonstick saucepan and bring to a boil. Turn off heat and stir in ramen noodles, sesame seeds, and almonds. Spoon the mixture onto prepared baking sheet and bake the crunchies until golden brown (do not burn) for about 22 minutes, turning every 8 minutes. Remove pan from oven and let crunchies cool.

4. To make the dressing, bring vinegar, canola oil, corn syrup, soy sauce, and remaining ramen soup broth powder to a boil in small nonstick saucepan. Boil 1 minute, remove pan from heat, and let cool.

5. Drizzle dressing over cabbage mixture and toss. Sprinkle the crunchies over the top and serve immediately (the crunchies will get soggy over time).

Nutritional Facts (*per serving*): 321 calories, 13 g protein, 32 g carbohydrate, 18 g fat (2.8 g saturated fat, 8.5 g monounsaturated fat, 5.7 g polyunsaturated fat, 1 g omega-3 fatty acids, 4.7 g omega-6 fatty acids), 5 mg cholesterol, 7 g fiber, 392 mg sodium. **Calories from fat: 50 percent.**

81 RE vitamin A, 69 mg vitamin C, 1.3 IU vitamin D, 6 IU vitamin E, 0 mcg vitamin B_{12}, 139 mcg folate, 233 mg calcium, 11 mcg selenium.

Cinnamon Rolls with Soy Flour

Lots of people look forward to those ooey, gooey cinnamon rolls when they go to the mall. This is a lighter version you can make at home with your bread machine.

Makes 12 rolls • Serving size: one roll

DOUGH:

1 cup plus 2 tablespoons warm lowfat milk (105–110 degrees)

3 tablespoons melted butter or no- or low-trans-fat margarine (for example, Land O' Lakes Fresh Buttery Taste Spread or Smart Balance)

1 egg, lightly beaten

¼ cup egg substitute

½ cup sugar

3 cups unbleached flour

1 cup soy flour

1 teaspoon salt

4 teaspoons active dry yeast

FILLING:

1 cup packed brown sugar

2 tablespoons ground cinnamon

¼ cup diet margarine (such as I Can't Believe It's Not Butter Margarine Light, Land O' Lakes Fresh Buttery Taste Spread, or Smart Balance)

ICING (OPTIONAL):

½ cup soy cream cheese (ie., Veggie Cream
Cheese by Galaxy Nutritional Foods)
2 tablespoons butter or diet margarine,
softened

1½ cups powdered sugar
½ teaspoon vanilla extract

1. Place dough ingredients in a 2-pound bread machine in the order recommended by the manufacturer. Set machine to the dough cycle and press start.
2. When the dough cycle is complete, roll dough out on a lightly floured surface until it is about 21 inches long and 16 inches wide. It should be about ¼ inch thick.
3. Combine the brown sugar and cinnamon in a bowl. Spread the diet margarine evenly over the surface of the dough, and then sprinkle the cinnamon mixture evenly over the margarine.
4. Working carefully from the 21-inch side, roll the dough down to the bottom edge. Cut the rolled dough into 1¾-inch slices and place in a single layer in a 9x13-inch pan that has been coated with canola oil cooking spray. You can cover the slices and let them rise in the refrigerator overnight, or let them rise at room temperature for an hour.
5. Bake in a preheated 400-degree oven for about 10 minutes, or until the rolls are light brown on top and cooked throughout. While the rolls bake, beat the icing ingredients with an electric mixer until fluffy. When the rolls come out of the oven, coat each generously with icing.

Nutritional Facts: 392 calories, 9 g protein, 70 g carbohydrate, 9 g fat (3.3 g saturated fat, 1.1 g monounsaturated fat, 0.3 g polyunsaturated fat, 0.1 g omega-3 fatty acids, 0.2 g omega-6 fatty acids), 30 mg cholesterol, 2.5 g fiber, 349 mg sodium. Calories from fat: 21 percent.

130 RE vitamin A, 0.2 mg vitamin C, 15 IU vitamin D, 0.3 IU vitamin E, 0.2 mcg vitamin B$_{12}$, 85 mcg folate, 74 mg calcium, 13 mcg selenium.

County Fair Cornbread with Soy Flour

Most people won't be able to tell that these muffins contain some soy flour. The yellow color from the cornmeal hides the yellowish tint from the soy flour well.

Makes 16 corn muffins • Serving size: 1 muffin

½ cup white sugar

1 teaspoon salt

¼ cup butter or no-trans-fat margarine, softened

1 teaspoon vanilla extract

1 large egg

¼ cup egg substitute

1 cup white flour

½ cup whole-wheat flour

½ cup soy flour

1 tablespoon baking powder

¾ cup cornmeal

6 tablespoons lowfat buttermilk

1 cup lowfat milk

1. Preheat oven to 400 degrees. Line a cupcake or muffin pan with muffin papers.
2. In large mixing bowl, beat sugar, salt, butter or margarine, and vanilla extract together until creamy. Beat in egg and egg substitute on medium-low speed.
3. In separate bowl, mix together flours, baking powder, and cornmeal. Beat flour mixture into egg mixture alternately with buttermilk and milk on low speed. Beat only until blended.
4. Fill each muffin cup with about ¼ cup of batter and bake for 20 minutes or until golden brown. Serve warm.

Nutritional Facts *(per muffin)*: 142 calories, 4.5 g protein, 22 g carbohydrate, 4.2 g fat (2 g saturated fat, 1 g monounsaturated fat, 0.3 g polyunsaturated fat, 0.1 g omega-3 fatty acids, 0.2 g omega-6 fatty acids), 22 mg cholesterol, 2 g fiber, 275 mg sodium. Calories from fat: 27 percent.

45 RE vitamin A, 0 mg vitamin C, 11 IU vitamin D, 0.3 IU vitamin E, 0.1 mcg vitamin B_{12}, 29 mcg folate, 80 mg calcium, 7 mcg selenium.

Soy Soft Pretzels

Somehow the freshly made pretzels at the mall taste so much better than anything you've made at home. But this recipe will get you really close to mall pretzels. You can top them with salt or cinnamon sugar, or you can get fancy and dip them in cheese sauce, mustard, or pizza sauce. The best part is, these homemade pretzels have a dose of soy flour in them! This recipe requires one rising period of about one hour.

Makes 12 pretzels • Serving size: 1 pretzel

1¼ cups very warm water	1 tablespoon canola oil
1 teaspoon sugar	1 tablespoon dark corn syrup or molasses
4 teaspoons active dry yeast	½ cup baking soda
4 cups all-purpose flour	4 cups hot water from tap
1 cup soy flour	⅓ cup kosher salt, for topping
⅓ cup granulated sugar	2 tablespoons melted butter
1½ teaspoons salt	

1. Add 1¼ cups warm water and 1 teaspoon sugar to a 2-cup measure. Sprinkle yeast over the top and let stand until creamy, about 10 minutes.
2. In a mixing bowl, blend flours, ⅓ cup sugar, and salt on low speed. Form a well in the center and add the canola oil, corn syrup, and yeast mixture. Beat on lowest speed to form a dough. If mixture is dry, add a couple more tablespoons of water.
3. Knead dough on a flat surface that has been generously dusted with flour about 6 minutes, until smooth. Lightly oil a large bowl with canola oil, then place the dough in the bowl and turn to coat with oil. Cover with plastic wrap and let rise in a warm place until doubled in size, about 1 hour, or overnight in the refrigerator.
4. Preheat oven to 450 degrees. In a large bowl, dissolve baking soda in 4 cups hot water. When dough is ready, turn out onto the lightly floured surface and divide into 12 equal pieces. Roll each piece into a rope and twist into a pretzel shape. When all the dough is shaped, dip each pretzel into the baking soda solution and place on a greased baking sheet. Sprinkle each pretzel with kosher salt.
5. Bake in oven until browned (about 8 minutes). Brush the tops of warm pretzels with melted butter. Sprinkle with additional salt if desired.

Nutritional Facts (*per pretzel*): 242 calories, 8 g protein, 42 g carbohydrate, 5 g fat (1.6 g saturated fat, 1.3 g monounsaturated fat, 0.6 g polyunsaturated fat, 0.2 g omega-3 fatty acids, 0.4 g omega-6 fatty acids), 5 mg cholesterol, 3 g fiber, 315 mg sodium. Calories from fat: 18 percent.

18 RE vitamin A, 0 mg vitamin C, 1.3 IU vitamin D, 0.5 IU vitamin E, 0 mcg vitamin B_{12}, 95 mcg folate, 22 mg calcium, 15 mcg selenium.

Wheat and Soy Bread

If you have a bread machine in the back of your kitchen cupboard, it's time to dust it off! This is a nice wheat bread made with whole-wheat flour, unbleached white flour and soy flour.

Makes 12 slices (1 9x5-inch loaf) • *Serving size: 1 slice*

1 cup warm water	*1¼ cups whole-wheat flour*
¼ cup sugar	*1 cup unbleached white flour*
1 tablespoon canola oil	*¾ cup soy flour (whole-grain)*
1 tablespoon fat-free sour cream	*1 tablespoon active dry yeast*
* or lowfat yogurt*	*½ teaspoon salt*

1. Add water, sugar, canola oil, sour cream, and flours to bread machine pan. Make a well in the center of the flour and add the yeast. Add the salt to a corner of the bread machine pan.

2. Set bread machine to Dough cycle and press start.

3. When the dough cycle is complete (about 1 hour and 40 minutes), press dough into a 9x5-inch pan coated with canola cooking oil spray. Allow the dough to rise for 30 minutes or until it has risen 1 inch above the pan. Preheat oven to 350 degrees.

4. Bake for about 30 minutes or until cooked throughout.

Nutritional Facts (*per serving*): 132 calories, 5 g protein, 23 g carbohydrate, 2.5 g fat, (0.3 g saturated fat, 1 g monounsaturated fat, 1.1 g polyunsaturated fat, 0.8 mg omega-3 fatty acids, 0.3 g omega-6 fatty acids), 0 mg cholesterol, 2.1 g fiber, 91 mg sodium. Calories from fat: 17 percent.

3 RE vitamin A, 0 mg vitamin C, 0 vitamin D, 0.4 IU vitamin E, 0 B_{12}, 40 mcg folate, 19 mg calcium, 13 mcg selenium.

Creamy Pesto Pasta Surprise

The "creamy" and "surprise" parts of this recipe's name have to do with one ingredient—silken (soft) light tofu. If you don't tell your family this recipe is made with tofu, they'll never know it. You can serve this dish with slices of roasted turkey, chicken, shrimp, or lean sliced chicken-sausage links. The carrots not only add color, they add two types of phyto-estrogens—isoflavonoids and lignans. *Makes 2 servings • Serving size: about 2 cups*

3 tablespoons store-bought or homemade pesto (I like to use Armanino Farms from the frozen-food section)
½ cup silken (soft) light tofu
¼ cup reduced-fat Monterey Jack cheese or part-skim mozzarella, grated (packed measure)

3 cups cooked spaghetti noodles
1 cup julienne carrots, cut into thin 2-inch long strips or thinly siced on the diagonal
Freshly shredded Parmesan cheese to taste (optional)

1. In a small food processor or small mixing bowl, blend pesto, tofu, and grated cheese together until creamy and fairly smooth.
2. Place about half of the cooked noodles on each plate or in individual pasta bowls. Spread half the pesto cream sauce over the top of each serving of noodles, then sprinkle carrots evenly over the top.
3. Cover and microwave each plate/bowl on high power for about 3 minutes, or until the pasta is nice and hot and the carrots are lightly tender. Sprinkle Parmesan over the top if desired. Serve!

Nutritional Facts *(per serving)*: 474 calories, 21 g protein, 70 g carbohydrate, 12 g fat (3.5 g saturated fat, 0.3 g monounsaturated fat, 1 g polyunsaturated fat, 0.1 g omega-3 fatty acids, 0.6 g omega-6 fatty acids), 14 mg cholesterol, 6.3 g fiber, 360 mg sodium. Calories from fat: 23 percent.

2122 RE vitamin A, 6 mg vitamin C, 0 IU vitamin D, 1 IU vitamin E, 0.1 mcg vitamin B_{12}, 157 mcg folate, 229 mg calcium, 45 mcg selenium.

Note: If you happen to have some of the tofu pesto sauce left over, it makes a wonderful filling for stuffed mushroom appetizers. Just spoon the sauce into mushroom caps and bake or microwave them until the mushrooms are tender. Then put the mushrooms under the broiler and broil just until the pesto is lightly browned.

Chicken Lettuce Wraps
with Crunchy Soynuts

This is a fun entrée or appetizer that you can eat with your hands. The crisp and cold lettuce makes it a pleasantly cool but still savory entrée. I suggest a 30-minute marinating time for the chicken in this recipe. *Makes 8 wraps • Serving size: 1 wrap*

2 teaspoons light soy sauce

4 teaspoons dry sherry (chicken broth can be substituted)

1 teaspoon sesame oil

1 teaspoon cornstarch

2 large (or 3 small) boneless, skinless chicken breasts

2 teaspoons canola oil

1 tablespoon minced or chopped garlic (about 4 large cloves)

1 tablespoon finely chopped fresh ginger

3 green onions (white and part of green), chopped

½ cup finely chopped or grated carrot (about 1 carrot)

½ cup finely chopped celery (about 1 small stalk)

2 tablespoons bottled hoisin sauce (can be found in the Asian food section of supermarket)

2 tablespoons bottled plum sauce (can be found in the Asian food section of supermarket)

8 large leaves of iceberg lettuce

½ –¾ cup toasted soynuts

1. Mix soy sauce, sherry, sesame oil, and cornstarch in a 2-cup measure.
2. Place chicken breasts in a food processor. Drizzle the marinade over the top and process mixture until chicken looks like ground pork. Cover container and refrigerate at least 30 minutes.
3. Heat nonstick wok or skillet on medium heat. Add canola oil, garlic, and ginger, and cook 30 seconds. Add chicken mixture, breaking chunks into small pieces until cooked through. Add chopped vegetables; toss for 1 minute or until tender-crisp. Stir in hoisin and plum sauces; toss to mix.
4. Spoon ⅛ of the mixture into the center of each lettuce leaf, sprinkle a heaping tablespoon of soynuts over the chicken mixture, roll up slightly, and serve!

Nutritional Facts (*per serving*): 134 calories, 15 g protein, 8.5 g carbohydrate, 4.3 g fat (0.8 g saturated fat, 1.2 g monounsaturated fat, 0.7 g polyunsaturated fat, 0.2 g omega-3 fatty acids, 0.6 g omega-6 fatty acids), 30 mg cholesterol, 2.2 g fiber, 171 mg sodium. Calories from fat: 29 percent.

203 RE vitamin A, 3 mg vitamin C, 4 IU vitamin D, 0.7 IU vitamin E, 0.1 mcg vitamin B$_{12}$, 16 mcg folate, 35 mg calcium, 0.10 mcg selenium.

Coconut Curried Tofu with Vegetables

This colorful curry dish features a medley of vegetables and a hint of coconut and cream for an exotic Thai treat. Serve over cooked brown rice to make it a complete meal.

Makes 4 servings • Serving size: about 2 cups

2–4 cups cooked brown rice

½ cup fat-free half-and-half

1 teaspoon coconut extract

1 tablespoon canola oil

16 ounces extra-firm tofu, drained, patted dry, and cut into 1 x 2-inch triangles

½ cup green onions, thinly sliced

1 teaspoon curry powder (or more to taste)

1 teaspoon ground cumin

⅛ teaspoon crushed red pepper flakes (optional)

2 teaspoons fresh ginger, minced

1 teaspoon garlic, minced or chopped

1 cup bite-size broccoli florets, lightly microwaved or steamed

1 cup carrots, sliced at a diagonal, lightly microwaved or steamed

2 tablespoons roasted peanuts, chopped (optional)

1. Cook the brown rice according to the directions on the package. Pour half-and-half into 1-cup measure and stir in the coconut extract; set aside.

2. Heat canola oil in a large nonstick skillet over high heat. Add tofu triangles and stir-fry until golden, about 6 minutes. Add green onions, curry powder, cumin, red pepper if desired, ginger, and garlic, and stir-fry a minute or two more.

3. Stir in broccoli florets, carrot slices, and half-and-half/coconut mixture. Reduce heat to simmer and let the mixture cook, covered, for 2 minutes. Season with salt and pepper if desired.

4. Serve tofu mixture over a small mound of brown rice. Sprinkle each serving with chopped peanuts if desired.

Nutritional Facts (*per serving*): 300 calories, 17 g protein, 35 g carbohydrate, 11.5 g fat (1.5 g saturated fat, 4 g monounsaturated fat, 5.3 g polyunsaturated fat, 0.8 g omega-3 fatty acids, 4.5 g omega-6 fatty acids), 0 mg cholesterol, 4.5 g fiber, 73 mg sodium. Calories from fat: 34 percent.

1,068 RE vitamin A, 23 mg vitamin C, 24 IU vitamin D, 2.3 IU vitamin E, 0 mcg vitamin B_{12}, 59 mcg folate, 236 mg calcium, 20 mcg selenium.

Oven-Baked Tempeh (or Tofu)

If you can't find tempeh in your local grocery store, using firm tofu works well too. Serve this dish over cooked brown rice or with some whole grain crackers or toast if desired.

Makes 6 servings • Serving size: about 1 cup

1½ teaspoons olive oil

⅛ teaspoon crushed red pepper flakes

1 leek, sliced (white and part of the green)

⅓ cup shallots, chopped

⅔ cup red bell pepper, chopped

4 cloves garlic, minced (about 1 tablespoon)

2 cups baby carrots, halved

1 cup zucchini, diced

1 8-ounce package seasoned tempeh (or use a 12-ounce firm tofu block cut into about 9 slices, 1 centimeter thick)

½ cup dry sherry (chicken broth can be substituted)

2 tomatoes, chopped

1 tablespoon tamari (or 2 tablespoons reduced-sodium soy sauce)

1. Preheat oven to 350 degrees.
2. Place oil, red pepper flakes, leek, shallots, red pepper, and garlic in a large nonstick saucepan. Sauté for 3 minutes. Add the carrots, zucchini, and tempeh or tofu slices, and sauté, stirring frequently, for 5 minutes. Add the sherry, tomatoes, and tamari, and sauté for an additional 5 minutes.
3. Spoon mixture into a 9x13-inch baking dish, cover with foil, and bake in a 350-degree oven for 30 minutes. Serve!

Nutritional Facts (*per serving*): 152 calories, 10 g protein, 21 g carbohydrate, 2.5 g fat (0.5 g saturated fat, 0.9 g monounsaturated fat, 0.3 g polyunsaturated fat, 0.1 g omega-3 fatty acids, 0.2 g omega-6 fatty acids), 0 mg cholesterol, 5.6 g fiber, 233 mg sodium. Calories from fat: 15 percent.

1,478 RE vitamin A, 52 mg vitamin C, 0 IU vitamin D, 1.3 IU vitamin E, 0 mcg vitamin B_{12}, 38 mcg folate, 46 mg calcium, 0.8 mcg selenium.

Smoked Tofu—Broccoli Burrito

Sounds too healthy to be good—doesn't it? But it really tastes great and it's one of my favorite lunches.

Makes 1 large Burrito • Serving size: 1 Burrito

½ teaspoon canola oil
½ cup broccoli florets, coarsely chopped
⅛ cup onion, chopped
⅛ cup mushroom, chopped
1 small block (about 6.5 ounces) smoked or hickory-flavored baked tofu, diced
1 ounce reduced-fat Monterey Jack, garlic-flavored Monterey Jack cheese, or other reduced-fat cheese, shredded

½ cup cooked brown rice
1 large tortilla (whole-wheat and higher-fiber tortillas are now available in many supermarkets)

1. Add canola oil, broccoli, onion, and mushrooms to a small nonstick frying pan and sauté until just tender, about 3 minutes.
2. Stir in tofu and sauté together a minute or two more. Stir in the cheese and brown rice until the cheese is melted. Remove from heat.
3. Add the filling down the center of a large tortilla and wrap up like a burrito. Enjoy!

Note: You can buy instant brown rice that is now available and follow the directions on the box, using your microwave, and you'll have brown rice in 10 minutes.

Nutritional Facts *(per serving):* 384 calories, 22 g protein, 51 g carbohydrate, 10.5 g fat (4 g saturated fat, 3 g monounsaturated fat, 3.5 g polyunsaturated fat, 0.6 g omega-3 fatty acids, 3.3 g omega-6 fatty acids), 20 mg cholesterol, 6 g fiber, 430 mg sodium. Calories from fat: 25 percent.

188 RE vitamin A, 36 mg vitamin C, 6.4 IU vitamin D, 2.7 IU vitamin E, 0.3 mcg vitamin B_{12}, 100 mcg folate, 383 mg calcium, 0.23 mcg selenium.

Vegetable and Tofu Noodle Stir-Fry

This recipe packs a vegetable wallop, what with half a head of cabbage and cauliflower, three carrots, and two onions. Split four ways, each serving ends up offering 8 grams of fiber, a day's worth of vitamin C (93 mg), a good dose of vitamin A (380 RE), and almost 90 percent of the U.S. RDA for folic acid (157 mcg), among scores of phytochemicals and other vitamins and minerals.

Makes 4 large servings • Serving size: about 4 cups

2 (3-ounce) packages chicken or pork ramen noodles and 1 of the seasoning packets

1½ tablespoons canola oil

½ medium cauliflower head (cut away the core and cut the rest into florets)

3 carrots, thinly sliced

1 block firm tofu, diced

2 medium onions, peeled and quartered, then sliced

½ small head cabbage, thinly sliced

2 tablespoons light soy sauce

1 teaspoon sesame oil

1. Cook ramen noodles in medium saucepan according to the package directions, then drain well. Add back to saucepan and sprinkle the seasoning over the top of noodles and stir to blend; set aside.

2. Heat canola oil in heavy, large nonstick skillet over medium heat. Add cauliflower, carrots, tofu, and onions. Cover skillet and cook, stirring frequently, until crisp-tender (about 6–8 minutes).

3. Spread cabbage over the top of vegetables, stir into vegetables, cover pan, and continue to cook, stirring frequently, until cabbage is softened (about 3 minutes). Remove from heat. Mix in cooked noodles, soy sauce, and sesame oil, and serve!

Nutritional Facts *(per serving)*: 337 calories, 21 g protein, 37 g carbohydrate, 14 g fat (1.7 g saturated fat, 4.7 g monounsaturated fat, 5.8 g polyunsaturated fat, 1.2 g omega-3 fatty acids, 4.7 g omega-6 fatty acids), 0 mg cholesterol, 8 fiber, 560 mg sodium. Calories from fat: 37 percent.

380 RE vitamin A, 93 mg vitamin C, 0 IU vitamin D, 2.1 IU vitamin E, 0 mcg vitamin B$_{12}$, 157 mcg folate, 225 mg calcium, 15 mcg selenium.

Banana Coffee Cake with Chocolate-Chip Streusel

You can freeze servings of this coffee cake and use the microwave at home or at work to thaw it for a quick mid-morning or afternoon snack! This is a very painless way to work some ground flaxseeds into your day.

Makes 12 snack-size servings • Serving size: one piece, 2 inches by 2½ inches

¾ cup mini semisweet chocolate chips

½ cup dark brown sugar, packed

⅓ cup chopped pecans or walnuts

2 teaspoons ground cinnamon

6 tablespoons ground flaxseeds

1 cup whole-wheat pastry flour

½ cup white flour

¾ teaspoon baking soda

¾ teaspoon baking powder

¼ teaspoon salt

½ cup granulated sugar

¼ cup no-trans-fat margarine (butter can also be used), softened

1 large egg

1⅓ cups very ripe bananas (about 3 large bananas), mashed

¼ cup plus 3 tablespoons lowfat buttermilk

1. Preheat oven to 350 degrees. Coat an 8x8x2-inch baking dish with canola oil cooking spray.

2. For the streusel, add chocolate chips, brown sugar, pecans, cinnamon, and flaxseeds to a small bowl and stir with a whisk until well blended; set aside.

3. Add whole-wheat and white flours, baking soda, baking powder, and salt to medium bowl and stir with whisk until blended.

4. Add sugar, margarine, and egg to another mixing bowl and beat on medium speed until fluffy, scraping sides of bowl at least once. Beat in bananas and buttermilk and blend well. Slowly add dry ingredients to mixing bowl and beat on low until blended.

5. Spread half the batter in a prepared baking dish and sprinkle with half the streusel. Spread the remaining batter on top and top with remaining streusel. Bake coffee cake until tester inserted in center comes out clean, about 45–55 minutes.

Nutritional Facts *(per serving)*: 280 calories, 5 g protein, 43 g carbohydrate, 11 g fat (3 g saturated fat, 4.7 g monounsaturated fat, 3 g polyunsaturated fat, 0.8 g omega-3 fatty acids, 1.1 g omega-6 fatty acids), 18 mg cholesterol, 4 g fiber, 205 mg sodium. Calories from fat: 35 percent.

44 RE vitamin A, 2.4 mg vitamin C, 12 IU vitamin D, 1 IU vitamin E, 0 mcg vitamin B$_{12}$, 32 mcg folate, 54 mg calcium, 11 mcg selenium.

3.

Who Poured a Bucket of Water over

Me While I Was Sleeping?

Recipes to Minimize Night Sweats

Ever wake up at night smack-dab in the middle of what seems to be a puddle of perspiration? Twenty-five to forty percent of menopausal women have night-sweat episodes.

Aren't night sweats just hot flashes that hit while we're asleep? Maybe, maybe not. It's still being debated. The big difference is that with a night sweat, the emphasis is on the "sweat" part: You are excessively sweating rather than "flashing." That said, it still makes sense to follow the food and lifestyle hints in Chapter 2 to discourage hot flashes if you are trying to decrease night sweats.

You might also want to give the following food and lifestyle hints a go as well. You have nothing to lose and a good night's sleep to gain.

- Keep your bedroom temperature on the cool side at night. If you don't already have a ceiling fan above your bed, you might want to make the investment.
- Avoid those hot-flash trigger foods and drinks before bedtime (see page 14).

- Take a long, cool bath or shower before bed to bring your body temperature down right before you begin your slumber.
- Get into the exercise groove. Regular exercise encourages deeper, more productive sleep—and with night sweats, that's a good thing. You may still sweat, but you may not wake up because of it!

Recipes to Cool Off By

In this chapter, we are aiming for cool recipes to help lower your body temperature before bedtime (or during the day), and at the same time (whenever possible) incorporating some high-phytoestrogen fruits while we're at it. I've also thrown in a pasta salad with phyto-estrogen-rich ingredients for a cool, light dinner.

Frozen Fruit Freeze

Pick your favorite frozen fruit and blend it with some lowfat yogurt and a packet of sweetener (if you desire), and you've got a quick, made-to-order sorbet. The ground flaxseeds can be stirred in or blended in for a daily dose of phytoestrogens.

Makes 1 serving • Serving size: about 1⅓ cups

1 6-ounce carton lowfat vanilla yogurt
⅔ cup of your favorite frozen fruit (boysenberries are my favorite)

1 packet Splenda (optional)
1 tablespoon ground flaxseeds

1. Add yogurt and boysenberries (and Splenda if desired) to a blender or food processor and pulse until combined well.
2. Add to a serving dish and stir in flaxseeds.

Nutritional Facts (*per serving*): 228 calories, 11 g protein, 37 g carbohydrate, 5 g fat (1.6 g saturated fat, 1.2 g monounsaturated fat, 2 g polyunsaturated fat, 1.5 g omega-3 fatty acids, 0.5 g omega-6 fatty acids), 8 mg cholesterol, 6 g fiber, 116 mg sodium. Calories from fat: 20 percent.

28 RE vitamin A, 5 mg vitamin C, 3 IU vitamin D, 1.3 IU vitamin E, 1 mcg vitamin B_{12}, 97 mcg folate, 331 mg calcium, 9.3 mcg selenium.

Hot Flash Mochaccino

While a hot cup of caffeinated coffee will encourage a hot flash, this beverage will help chill your hot flash and keep you calm—and it will even slide a serving of phytoestrogen-rich soymilk into your day. If you would like, you can stir in a tablespoon of ground flaxseeds which will boost your fiber, phytoestrogens, and plant-derived omega-3 fatty acid totals too. For a variation, try caramel syrup instead of chocolate, and use plain or vanilla soymilk.

Makes 1 drink • Serving size: about 2 cups

*½ cup double-strength decaf coffee,
    chilled*

¾ cup chocolate soymilk

1½ cups ice cubes

*1 tablespoon ground flaxseeds
    (optional)*

*1 tablespoon chocolate syrup
    (optional)*

1. Add coffee, chocolate soymilk, ice cubes, and flaxseeds (if desired) into the blender and blend until the mixture has a nice, smooth texture (like a milkshake).
2. Taste the drink. If you would like a stronger chocolate flavor, add a tablespoon of chocolate syrup. Blend the mixture, pour into a tall glass, and enjoy!

Note: *If you don't have a blender, just mix the first 2 ingredients (and chocolate syrup, if desired) together, stir in the flaxseeds (if desired), and then add ice.*

Nutritional Facts (per serving without optional ingredients): 110 calories, 4 g protein, 18 g carbohydrate, 2.6 g fat (n/a g saturated fat, n/a g monounsaturated fat, n/a g polyunsaturated fat, n/a g omega-3 fatty acids, n/a g omega-6 fatty acids), 0 mg cholesterol, 0 g fiber, 61 mg sodium. Calories from fat: 21 percent.

75 RE vitamin A, 0 mg vitamin C, 90 IU vitamin D, 0 IU vitamin E, 2.3 mcg vitamin B_{12}, 18 mcg folate, 230 mg calcium, n/a mcg selenium.

Malted Strawberry Milk Shake

Make this shake when you need something sinful and sweet. The strawberries and flaxseeds give you some phytoestrogens, and the ice cream will help cool you off.

Makes 2 servings • Serving size: about 1½ cups each

½ cup lowfat milk

3 tablespoons malted-milk powder

1½ cups light vanilla ice cream or frozen
  yogurt

1 cup sliced strawberries, firmly packed

2 tablespoons ground flaxseeds

1–2 tablespoons strawberry syrup,
  (optional)

Malted milk balls, cut in half (optional)

1. Place milk, malt powder, vanilla ice cream, strawberries, flaxseeds, and strawberry syrup in a blender and process until well blended (you can add an extra tablespoon or two of milk if you like your shake a little thinner).

2. Pour into 2 cups, garnish each with a few malted milk ball halves if desired, and drink up with a straw or spoon.

Nutritional Facts *(per serving)*: 324 calories, 11 g protein, 51 g carbohydrate, 9.5 g fat (4 g saturated fat, 2.4 g monounsaturated fat, 2.5 g polyunsaturated fat, 1.7 g omega-3 fatty acids, 0.8 g omega-6 fatty acids), 24 mg cholesterol, 5 g fiber, 235 mg sodium. Calories from fat: 26 percent.

88 RE vitamin A, 49 mg vitamin C, 26 IU vitamin D, 1.1 IU vitamin E, 0.6 mcg vitamin B$_{12}$, 56 mcg folate, 295 mg calcium, 6 mcg selenium.

Shamrock Soy Shake

This flavorful shake requires a blender or food processor, but a mixer with a small bowl can be substituted.

Makes 1 serving • Serving size: 1 cup

½ cup lowfat vanilla frozen yogurt or
    light ice cream
½ cup soymilk (lowfat milk can also
    be used)

¹⁄₁₆ teaspoon mint extract
2 drops green food coloring
1–3 teaspoons ground flaxseeds if desired

1. Add all the ingredients to a blender and blend on medium speed until nice and smooth.
2. Pour into a short glass and serve with a spoon or straw.

Nutritional Facts (*per shake with 3 teaspoons ground flax*): 192 calories, 8 g protein, 23 g carbohydrate, 8.6 g fat (2.7 g saturated fat, 1.24 g monounsaturated fat, 1.16 g polyunsaturated fat), 15.6 mg cholesterol, 3.6 g fiber, 77 mg sodium. Calories from fat: 35 percent.

    31 RE vitamin A, 0.476 mg vitamin C, 0 IU vitamin D, 0.094 IU vitamin E, 0.51 mcg vitamin B$_{12}$, 3.84 mcg folate, 114 mg calcium, 3.1 mcg selenium.

Strawberry Crush Slush

Berries are good sources of isoflavones. You can stir in a teaspoon or two of ground flaxseeds if you want to add some of the other phytoestrogens (such as lignans), too.

Makes 1–2 servings • Serving size: 1 cup

1 cup crushed ice (or 1 heaping cup
    ice cubes)
2 tablespoons sugar
¾ cup sliced strawberries, firmly packed

⅓ cup diet lemon-lime soda (regular can
    be used if desired but will increase
    calories)

1. Add the ice, sugar, stawberries, and lemon-lime soda to a blender and pulse until it turns into a slush.
2. Pour into 2 glasses and serve with a straw or spoon.

Nutritional Facts (*per serving, if 2 servings per recipe*): 67 calories, 0.4 g protein, 17 g carbohydrate, 0.2 g fat (0 g saturated fat, 0 g monounsaturated fat, 0.1 g polyunsaturated fat, 0.05 g omega-3 fatty acids, 0.05 g omega-6 fatty acids), 0 mg cholesterol, 1.5 g fiber, 5 mg sodium. Calories from fat: 3 percent.

2 RE vitamin A, 35 mg vitamin C, 0 IU vitamin D, 0.2 IU vitamin E, 0 mcg vitamin B_{12}, 12 mcg folate, 9 mg calcium, 0.5 mcg selenium.

Strawberry Lemonade Smoothie

This recipe offers you a phytoestrogen-rich smoothie with a kick of calcium from the yogurt.   *Makes 1 smoothie • Serving size: about 1 1/2 cups*

1 cup frozen (unsweetened) whole
  strawberries, or 3/4 cup sliced
1/2 cup prepared sugar-free lemonade
  (like Crystal Lite)

1/2 cup lowfat lemon, vanilla,
  or plain yogurt
1 tablespoon ground flaxseeds

1. Add the ingredients to a blender or food processor and puree until well blended (about 1 minute).
2. Pour into a serving cup and add a straw!

Nutritional Facts (*per smoothie*): 190 calories, 9 g protein, 30 g carbohydrate, 4.8 g fat (1.3 g saturated fat, 1.1 g monounsaturated fat, 2 g polyunsaturated fat, 1.6 g omega-3 fatty acids, 0.5 g omega-6 fatty acids), 6 mg cholesterol, 6 g fiber, 85 mg sodium. Calories from fat: 23 percent.

21 RE vitamin A, 86 mg vitamin C, 2 IU vitamin D, 1 IU vitamin E, 0.7 mcg vitamin B_{12}, 62 mcg folate, 246 mg calcium, 8 mcg selenium.

Strawberry Sorbet in an Ice Cube Tray

No ice cream maker needed for this sorbet recipe! Just grab a blender and an ice cube tray and you are ready to refresh. This recipe offers not one but four sorbet flavors to cool you off on a hot summer night. It takes about 90 minutes to reach the right consistency in your freezer, so if you make it after dinner, it'll be sure to wet your whistle before bed.

Makes 1 ice cube tray of sorbet (about 4 servings) • Serving size: ½ cup

1 cup mashed strawberries, fresh or frozen

½ cup orange-strawberry juice or regular orange juice

½ cup sugar (Baker's superfine sugar works best)

1 teaspoon of ground flaxseeds per serving (optional)

1. Add the ingredients to a blender and pulse until blended well (or use an electric mixer).
2. Pour mixture into an ice cube tray. Freeze until mostly firm (1 hour or more).
3. Add about 4 sorbet cubes (to make one serving) to a small bowl and break up into a frozen slush-like mixture with a fork, or use a blender or food processor. Stir a teaspoon of flaxseeds into each serving if desired.

OTHER FLAVOR OPTIONS

For Peach-Mango Sorbet: substitute chopped peach slices (fresh, thawed frozen, or drained canned) for the strawberries, and mango-orange juice concentrate for the orange-strawberry juice.

For Go Grape Sorbet: substitute raspberries (fresh or thawed frozen) for the strawberries and grape juice concentrate for the orange-strawberry juice.

For Cherry Crush Sorbet: substitute pitted cherry halves (fresh, thawed frozen, or drained canned) for the strawberries and cherry juice concentrate or mixed berry juice concentrate for the orange-strawberry juice.

Note: *If you let your ice cubes freeze more than a few hours, they will be too hard to stir together with a spoon. In that case, just add all the ice cubes to a food processor and pulse for about 8 seconds to make the sorbet.*

Nutritional Facts *(per strawberry sorbet serving)*: 129 calories, 1 g protein, 32 g carbohydrate, 0.3 g fat (0.02 g saturated fat, 0.04 g monounsaturated fat, 0.13 g polyunsaturated fat, 0 g omega-3 fatty acids, 0 g omega-6 fatty acids), 0 mg cholesterol, 1 g fiber, 1.2 mg sodium. Calories from fat: 2 percent.

8 RE vitamin A, 51 mg vitamin C, 0 IU vitamin D, 0.1 IU vitamin E, 0 mcg vitamin B_{12}, 20 mcg folate, 12 mg calcium, 1 mcg selenium.

Pesto Pasta Salad

For something more substantial, here is a cool and light dinner (with phytoestrogen-rich ingredients) to help ease you into the late evening hours. If you have some diners who may not want tofu in their pasta salad, just divide the pasta salad into 2 serving bowls and add half the amount of tofu cubes to one of the bowls. Even people who don't care for tofu may like this dish, because the tofu can almost pass as a type of cheese—the texture works well. This salad also is great the next day as a lunch. *Makes 10 servings • Serving size: about 1½ cups*

12 ounces dry pasta noodles of choice. Using whole-wheat pasta will boost the fiber!

⅓ cup pine nuts

1 cup fresh basil, rinsed and drained well

2 cups vine-ripened tomatoes, chopped, or cherry tomatoes, quartered (orange and red cherry tomatoes can be used to give the salad even more color)

1 14-ounce can artichoke hearts, packed in water, drained. (If you use marinated artichoke hearts, rinse and drain well.)

1 container firm tofu (14 ounces drained weight), rinsed well and cut into ½-inch cubes

1 7-ounce container Armanino Pesto Sauce (in frozen food section of your supermarket) or 14 tablespoons of another pesto made with olive oil or canola oil, thawed

3 tablespoons grated Parmesan cheese

1. Prepare pasta according to package directions, boiling about 10–12 minutes, then drain well in colander.
2. While noodles are boiling, toast pine nuts in 400-degree oven (toast at 300 degrees if using a toaster oven) until light brown, watching carefully, about 3–5 minutes. You

can also toast them in a nonstick pan on the stove over medium heat. Cool and add to serving bowl.

3. Coarsely chop fresh basil; add to serving bowl. Chop tomatoes and artichoke hearts, and add with tofu to serving bowl.

4. Add drained noodles to serving bowl, along with pesto and Parmesan cheese, and toss everything together well. Serve or store in refrigerator until needed.

Nutritional Facts *(per serving)*: 245 calories, 10 g protein, 30 g carbohydrate, 9.5 g fat (2 g saturated fat, 1.5 g monounsaturated fat, 2.4 g polyunsaturated fat, 0.2 g omega-3 fatty acids, 1.8 g omega-6 fatty acids), 5 mg cholesterol, 3 g fiber, 163 mg sodium. Calories from fat: 35 percent.

121 RE vitamin A, 7 mg vitamin C, 0.4 IU vitamin D, 0.5 IU vitamin E, 0 mcg vitamin B_{12}, 71 mcg folate, 151 mg calcium, 5 mcg selenium.

4.

I'm So Tired.
Why Can't I Get to Sleep?

Diet Tips to Beat Insomnia

Many women find that the quality and quantity of their much-needed sleep seems to vanish along with their estrogen. Insomnia, defined as the inability to fall asleep or stay asleep at night, is a common side effect of menopause and is usually caused by other symptoms of menopause, such as hot flashes and night sweats.

I am not sleeping well at night.
Do I have insomnia?

Symptoms of insomnia can include one or more of the following:

- Difficulty falling asleep
- Waking up frequently during the night and having difficulty returning to sleep
- Waking up too early in the morning
- Non-refreshing sleep (feeling tired upon waking and throughout the day)

For women in the throes of menopause, it's the frequent awakenings, largely due to hot flashes and night sweats, and feeling tired after a night of sleep—or non-sleep, as the case may be—that seems to cause the problems.

Insomnia actually doesn't become a full-blown problem until it starts making you feel tired all the time. If you are less sleepy at night or wake up early but still feel rested and alert, you probably needn't worry too much about it.

But what if insomnia is bothering you and causing you to feel tired? The first thing you want to do is rule out other causes besides those related to menopause. Pay close attention to the information below about drinking caffeinated or alcoholic beverages later in the day. You might also want to review the information on night sweats in Chapter 3 if they are the main cause of your insomnia. Last, there are a few food and lifestyle tips you can try to promote higher-quality sleep.

Rule Out Other Causes of Insomnia

Occasional insomnia may be caused by noise, extreme temperatures, jet lag, changes in your sleep environment, a change in your sleep pattern, or temporary life stresses that come along every once in a while (such as work deadlines or a sickness or death in the family). This type of insomnia tends to disappear once you adjust to the life change or once the cause of your sleep problem goes away.

Long-term Insomnia

Long-term insomnia may last months or even years and may be caused by:

- **Anxiety.** If feelings of anxiety are causing your sleep problems, work with your health-care professional to develop a plan to decrease your anxiety and promote quality sleep.
- **Depression.** People who are depressed will usually have at least one of the following two symptoms:

  1. Feeling negative, hopeless, or always down in the dumps
  2. Noticeable loss of interest or pleasure in most activities

- **Other physical problems.** Asthma, coronary artery disease, or chronic obstructive pulmonary disease (COPD), a condition that makes it difficult to breathe because air does not flow easily out of the lungs, can be sources of insomnia.

Medications and Insomnia

Many medications, both prescription and nonprescription, can cause sleep problems. Take a moment to go through the lists below to help determine if your sleep problems could be caused or exacerbated by medications or social drugs you might be taking.

PRESCRIPTION MEDICATIONS THAT MAY
CAUSE SLEEP PROBLEMS INCLUDE:
- High-blood-pressure medications, including clonidine, propranolol, atenolol, and methyldopa.
- Hormones, such as oral contraceptives, thyroid medications, cortisone, and progesterone.
- Respiratory medications, such as theophylline, albuterol, and salmeterol.
- Steroids, such as prednisone and hexadrol.
- Other medications, such as diet pills, some antidepressants, attention deficit/hyperactivity disorder (ADHD) medications, phenytoin, levodopa, and quinidine.

NONPRESCRIPTION MEDICATIONS THAT MAY
CAUSE SLEEP PROBLEMS INCLUDE:
- Medications that contain caffeine, such as Anacin, Excedrin, Empirin, NoDoz, cough medicines, and cold medications.
- Pseudoephedrine, such as Sudafed.

SOCIAL DRUGS AND OTHER SUBSTANCES THAT MAY
CAUSE SLEEP PROBLEMS INCLUDE:
- Alcohol. Initially, drinking alcohol may cause sleepiness. Many people drink alcohol to help them go to sleep. However, you are likely to wake up just a few hours after going to sleep when the depressant effect of the alcohol wears off.
- Caffeine. Drinking a cup of coffee or other caffeine-containing beverage during the day can cause sleeplessness. Caffeine can stimulate the body for three to seven hours and can

interfere with your sleep as long as it remains in your body. Even the small amount of caffeine in decaffeinated beverages can interfere with sleep in particularly sensitive people.

- Nicotine can disrupt sleep and reduce total sleep time. Smokers report more daytime sleepiness and minor accidents than do nonsmokers, especially in younger age groups. Illegal drugs such as cocaine, amphetamines, and methamphetamines all can have a negative effect on sleep.

What lifestyle changes can I make to discourage insomnia?

To sleep soundly through the night, you might want to try the handful of lifestyle tips below. They certainly can't hurt, and they just may help.

- Do not nap during the day.
- Exercise daily. However, be sure to avoid vigorous exercise within three hours of bedtime. Exercising late at night tends to stimulate your body in many ways, giving you a second wind when your body should be winding down.
- Avoid stimulants such as caffeine, alcohol, and nicotine throughout the entire day.
- Keep your bedroom cool to prevent night sweats.
- Do not go to bed until you are tired. There's nothing worse than trying so hard to go to sleep that you get more and more anxious as time passes. The more anxious you get about not falling asleep, the further away slumberland becomes.
- Take a warm bath or shower at bedtime.
- Try to follow the same bedtime routine each night. Your body will hopefully find comfort and rhythm in these nighttime rituals.
- Avoid using sleeping pills and other medications that promote insomnia.

How to Eat to Sleep

What can we eat (or not eat) to help us sleep better? The first place to start adjusting your food choices to promote sleep is at dinnertime. What do many people usually do at dinnertime? They eat large meals featuring a giant serving of a high-protein meat. If this describes your dinner routine, you could be going about it all wrong. Instead, to help you sleep better, try including the following foods in your evening meal, recommends Judith Wurtman, Ph.D., director of a women's health program at MIT Clinical Research Center in Boston.

- potatoes
- pasta
- couscous
- vegetables
- beans and rice

What do all of the above foods have in common? Carbs, carbs, and more carbs. Dr. Wurtman suggests that in order to prevent insomnia, your dinner should be pretty much vegetarian. Eating carbs and little to no protein for dinner increases serotonin synthesis, which can make you feel calmer in the evening, which may help promote sleep. (Serotonin is a chemical in the brain that helps control sleep patterns, appetite, pain, and other functions.)

Will drinking warm milk help me fall asleep?

Milk contains a substance called tryptophan. The body uses tryptophan to make serotonin. Sounds good so far, doesn't it? Unfortunately, milk doesn't contain enough tryptophan to actually change your sleep patterns. However, drinking a glass of milk before bed may simply help you relax—which may indirectly contribute to a better night's sleep.

Melatonin Supplements

Women who find themselves waking up several times during the night could try a preparation of 0.3 mg melatonin, Dr. Wurtman says. This is the amount of melatonin that will correct any age-related decrease in the amount of melatonin your body makes. But don't think that if 0.3 mg is good, 0.6 mg must be better—Dr. Wurtman also warns menopausal women that if doses are higher than 0.3 mg, the melatonin will stop working within a few days and can cause side effects such as hyperthermia and drowsiness.

Fight Fatigue with Food

Mild fatigue can often be prevented by changes in the following lifestyle habits.

- Eat a well-balanced diet. Do not skip meals—especially breakfast.
- Make sure you are getting enough good-quality fuel (food calories) for energy—which requires eating a healthy diet and drinking plenty of water.
- Start your day with a lowfat, high-fiber breakfast.
- Eat small-sized meals every three or so hours instead of eating large meals a couple times a day.
- Include fruits and vegetables, lean meats, or high-protein plant foods and lowfat dairy products in your meals and snacks throughout the day when possible. A morning or midday meal with some carbohydrate, fiber, protein, and fat is more likely to digest more slowly, providing the body with a more constant supply of energy.
- Don't fill up on high-fat or sugary foods—they tend to leave you feeling sluggish.
- Regular exercise is your best defense against fatigue. If you feel too tired to exercise vigorously, try taking a short walk.
- Make sure you are getting enough sleep.
- Deal with emotional problems instead of ignoring or denying them.
- Take steps to control your stress level and workload.

Sleep-Inducing Dinner Recipes

Creamy Hot Bean Dip

You can skip the cheese-grating step by buying a package of preshredded reduced-fat jack and cheddar cheese mixtures.

Makes 3½ cups • Serving size: ½ cup

½ cup (4 ounces) light cream cheese, softened at room temperature

½ cup fat-free or light sour cream

1 16-ounce can vegetarian or fat-free refried beans

1 tablespoon packaged taco seasoning mix

5 drops hot pepper sauce (such as Tabasco)

2 teaspoons dried parsley flakes

⅓ cup green onions (white and part of green), chopped

1 cup reduced-fat sharp cheddar cheese (4 ounces), shredded

1 cup reduced-fat Monterey Jack cheese (4 ounces), shredded

1. Preheat oven to 350 degrees. Coat an 8x8-inch baking dish or loaf pan with canola oil cooking spray.

2. In a mixing bowl, blend the cream cheese, sour cream, refried beans, taco seasoning, hot pepper sauce, parsley flakes, green onions, and half the cheese together on low speed (or stir by hand).

3. Spread mixture into prepared baking dish, sprinkle with remaining cheese, and bake at 350 degrees until bean dip is hot and cheese is bubbling, about 20 minutes.

Nutritional Facts *(per ½ cup serving)*: 211 calories, 14 g protein, 16 g carbohydrate, 10 g fat (6.7 g saturated fat, 1 g monounsaturated fat, 1 g polyunsaturated fat, 0 g omega-3 fatty acids, 0 g omega-6 fatty acids), 33 mg cholesterol, 3.5 g fiber, 743 mg sodium. Calories from fat: 42 percent.

163 RE vitamin A, 1 mg vitamin C, 0 IU vitamin D, 0 IU vitamin E, 0.2 mcg vitamin B_{12}, 3 mcg folate, 302 mg calcium, 0 mcg selenium.

Black Bean and Couscous Salad

This high-carb salad has a taste of the Southwest that you'll look forward to night after night. Leftovers store well, refrigerated, for several days.

Makes 8 servings • Serving size: about ¼ cup

1¼ cups low-sodium chicken or
    vegetable broth
1 cup uncooked couscous
3 tablespoons extra-virgin olive oil
2 tablespoons fresh lime juice
1 teaspoon red wine vinegar
½ teaspoon ground cumin

8 green onions, chopped
1 red or yellow bell pepper, seeded
    and finely chopped
¼ cup fresh cilantro, chopped
1 cup frozen corn kernels, thawed
2 15-ounce cans black beans, drained
Salt and pepper to taste

1. Bring broth to a boil in a 2-quart or larger saucepan and stir in the couscous. Cover the pot and remove from heat. Let stand for 5 minutes.
2. In a large bowl, whisk together the olive oil, lime juice, vinegar, and cumin. Add the green onions, pepper, cilantro, corn, and beans, and toss to coat.
3. Fluff the couscous well with a fork, breaking up any chunks. Add to the bowl with the vegetables and mix well. Season with salt and pepper to taste and serve at once or refrigerate until ready to serve.

Nutritional Facts *(per serving)*: 219 calories, 9 g protein, 37 g carbohydrate, 5.5 g fat (0.9 g saturated fat, 4.1 g monounsaturated fat, 0.6 g polyunsaturated fat, 0.1 g omega-3 fatty acids, 0.5 g omega-6 fatty acids), 1 mg cholesterol, 7.2 g fiber, 456 mg sodium. Calories from fat: 23 percent.

125 RE vitamin A, 45 mg vitamin C, 0 IU vitamin D, 1.2 IU vitamin E, 0 mcg vitamin B_{12}, 21 mcg folate, 49 mg calcium, 0.3 mcg selenium.

Spinach and Orzo Salad

This is a colorful and easy to make pasta salad that works great as a light dinner.

Makes 8 servings • Service size: 2 cups

1 16-ounce package uncooked orzo

1 10-ounce package baby spinach leaves, finely chopped

6 ounces reduced-fat feta cheese, crumbled (or 4 ounces of regular feta)

½ red onion, finely chopped

½ cup pine nuts, lightly browned on medium heat in toaster oven, oven, or in a nonstick frying pan

¼ cup fresh basil, finely chopped (1 teaspoon dried basil can be substituted)

¼ teaspoon ground white or black pepper (add more to taste)

3 tablespoons olive oil

¼ cup apple or pear juice

½ cup balsamic vinegar

1. Bring a large pot of lightly salted water to a boil. Add orzo and cook for 8 to 10 minutes or until al dente; drain and rinse with cold water.
2. Transfer pasta to a large bowl and stir in spinach, feta, onion, pine nuts, basil, and pepper. Toss with olive oil, juice, and balsamic vinegar.
3. Cover bowl and refrigerate until needed. Serve cold.

Nutritional Facts (*per serving*): 364 calories, 16 g protein, 49 g carbohydrate, 12.5 g fat (3.1 g saturated fat, 6 g monounsaturated fat, 2.4 g polyunsaturated fat, 0.2 g omega-3 fatty acids, 2.2 g omega-6 fatty acids), 8 mg cholesterol, 4 g fiber, 313 mg sodium. Calories from fat: 31 percent.

525 RE vitamin A, 13 mg vitamin C, 0 IU vitamin D, 2.5 IU vitamin E, 0 mcg vitamin B_{12}, 198 mcg folate, 94 mg calcium, 1.8 mcg selenium.

Sweet Pepper and Basil Pellet Pasta Salad

I used an entire box of the pellet pasta (which makes 7½ cups cooked) by Ronzoni called Acini di Pepe pasta. Pasta doesn't get much smaller than this, folks. I brought a big huge bowl of this salad to a BBQ and went home with an empty bowl—always a good sign.

Makes 10 servings • Serving size: 1 cup

1 16-ounce box Acini di Pepe Pasta
    (pasta pellets)

3 tablespoons olive oil

1 yellow bell pepper, seeded and finely
    chopped

1 orange or red bell pepper, seeded and
    finely chopped

1 red or yellow onion, chopped

1 tablespoon garlic, minced

1 teaspoon salt

½ teaspoon white pepper

2 teaspoons dried oregano flakes

1 cup loosely packed fresh basil leaves,
    coarsely chopped

1 small or ½ large lemon, cut into wedges

1. Boil pasta until just tender, according to directions on box, about 12 minutes. Draining this type of pasta can be tricky, since the pasta may be smaller than the size of the holes in your colander. You can either put some cheesecloth in your colander or use a fine-mesh strainer. Add the drained pasta to a large serving bowl and drizzle 2 tablespoons of olive oil over the top; toss to blend well.

2. Heat a large nonstick frying pan over medium heat and add the remaining tablespoon of olive oil. When hot, add the bell peppers, onion, and garlic, and sauté 5 minutes or until the mixture is just starting to brown, stirring frequently. About midway through the sautéing, sprinkle the salt, white pepper, and oregano flakes over the top and toss to blend. Let mixture cool completely.

3. Add pepper-onion mixture to pasta and toss to blend. Serve at room temperature or refrigerate until needed. (This recipe can all be prepared a day or two before a party or BBQ.)

4. Right before serving, add the fresh basil to the pasta mixture and squeeze the lemon wedges, drizzling their juice over the pasta. Toss to blend well. Add more salt and white pepper to taste, if desired.

Nutritional Facts (*per serving*): 210 calories, 7 g protein, 35 g carbohydrate, 5 g fat (0.8 g saturated fat, 3.3 g monounsaturated fat, 0.4 g polyunsaturated fat, 0.1 g omega-3 fatty acids, 0.3 g omega-6 fatty acids), 0 mg cholesterol, 2 g fiber, 235 mg sodium. Calories from fat: 21 percent.

220 RE vitamin A, 34 mg vitamin C, 0 IU vitamin D, 1 IU vitamin E, 0 mcg vitamin B_{12}, 104 mcg folate, 19 mg calcium, 0.2 mcg selenium.

Spaghetti with Puttanesca Sauce

When we hear the word "pasta," many of us automatically think of spaghetti. Well, this sauce is not your ordinary spaghetti sauce. It has all sorts of flavors going on, with ingredients like anchovy fillets, Greek olives, capers, and crushed red pepper flakes.

Makes 4 servings • Serving size: about 2 cups

2 tablespoons extra-virgin olive oil

1 tablespoon garlic, minced or chopped

1 28-ounce can Italian-style crushed tomatoes

4 anchovy filets, rinsed and finely chopped (about 1 ounce)

3 tablespoons tomato paste

2 tablespoons capers, drained

20 Greek or Spanish olives, pitted and coarsely chopped

¼ teaspoon crushed red pepper flakes (you can use more or less, depending on your preference)

8 ounces uncooked spaghetti noodles

Shredded or grated Parmesan cheese (optional)

1. Heat oil in a skillet over low heat. Add garlic, and sauté until golden (about 1–2 minutes). Add tomatoes with juice, and simmer 5 minutes.
2. Stir in anchovies, and then tomato paste. Add capers, olives, and red pepper flakes.
3. Simmer 10 minutes, stirring occasionally. While the sauce is simmering, cook spaghetti noodles in a large pot of boiling salted water according to directions on the package. Drain.
4. Toss noodles with sauce and serve immediately. Top with Parmesan cheese if desired.

Nutritional Facts (*per serving*): 397 calories, 12 g protein, 59 g carbohydrate, 14 g fat (1.9 g saturated fat, 9.5 g monounsaturated fat, 1.9 g polyunsaturated fat, 0.2 g omega-3 fatty acids, 1.2 g omega-6 fatty acids), 3 mg cholesterol, 7 g fiber, 1,070 mg sodium. Calories from fat: 31 percent.

172 RE vitamin A, 24 mg vitamin C, 2 IU vitamin D, 5 IU vitamin E, 0 mcg vitamin B_{12}, 127 mcg folate, 103 mg calcium, 34 mcg selenium.

Spicy Chicken Linguine

If you don't like spicy foods, you can still enjoy this wonderful dish—just use Mrs. Dash Extra Spicy instead of the crushed red pepper. This will give just enough spice for us "spice wimps." Then have some crushed red pepper at the table for those that would like to add it.

Makes 4 servings • Serving size: about 2½ cups

2 tablespoons butter

¼ cup fat-free or light sour cream

½ cup double-strength or concentrated chicken broth

1 medium onion, thinly sliced

1½ teaspoons garlic, minced or chopped

1 tablespoon dried basil leaves (or 2 teaspoons of dried Italian herbs)

½ teaspoon crushed red pepper (or 1 teaspoon Mrs. Dash Extra Spicy)

2 chicken boneless and skinless breasts, cut in half

1 10-ounce box frozen chopped spinach (thawed and squeezed gently of excess liquid)

3–4 cups cooked linguine, spaghetti, or angel-hair pasta

¾ cup shredded or grated Parmesan cheese

Salt and pepper to taste (optional)

1. Preheat oven to 350 degrees. Add butter to a 9x13-inch baking pan. Place pan in oven to melt butter (about 2 minutes). Remove from oven. Stir in the sour cream, using a fork. Slowly stir in the chicken broth. Then stir in the onion slices, garlic, basil, and crushed red pepper.

2. Coat both sides of the chicken breasts in the butter-spice mixture and spread them out evenly in the pan, placing some onion slices over each piece.

3. Cover the pan with foil and bake at 350 degrees for 45 minutes.

4. After chicken is cooked through, uncover the pan, lift out the chicken breasts, and place them temporarily on a plate. Then add the spinach, cooked pasta, and Parmesan to the pan, and toss to stir everything very well. Add salt and pepper to taste if desired.

5. Place chicken breasts on top of pasta and spinach mixture (sprinkle additional grated Parmesan cheese over the top if desired), and bake an additional 5–10 minutes. Serve!

Nutritional Facts *(per serving with ¾ cup noodles per serving):* 456 calories, 43 g protein, 40 g carbohydrate, 14 g fat (7.6 g saturated fat, 4.3 g monounsaturated fat, 1.5 g polyunsaturated fat, 0.3 g omega-3 fatty acids, 1.1 g omega-6 fatty acids), 101 mg cholesterol, 5 g fiber, 661 mg sodium. Calories from fat: 27 percent.

1,188 RE vitamin A, 20 mg vitamin C, 18 IU vitamin D, 1.9 IU vitamin E, 0.6 mcg vitamin B_{12}, 172 mcg folate, 342 mg calcium, 52 mcg selenium.

Pesto Sauce
(Frozen in an Ice Cube Tray)

I love this recipe, because it is a super-convenient way to make a quickie dinner with pasta and vegetables (two food items that some experts say help induce sleep). The trick is getting a few bunches of fresh basil when it's in season and whipping up some pesto sauce. You can freeze it in an ice-cube tray, transfer the cubes to a resealable freezer bag, and you'll be in business for the season.

Makes about 14–16 frozen pesto cubes (about 1½ cups of pesto sauce or 2½ cups of creamy pesto sauce, if you add a tablespoon of fat-free half-and-half for every cube of frozen sauce) Serving size: ⅛ cup

3 cups fresh basil leaves, rinsed, drained, and lightly packed into a measuring cup

6 tablespoons olive oil

1½–2 teaspoons garlic, minced

Juice from 1 lemon

⅓ cup toasted pine nuts (lightly brown nuts on medium heat in toaster oven or nonstick pan)

½ cup double-strength or concentrated chicken broth

½ cup shredded Parmesan cheese

1. Add all the ingredients to a food processor and pulse to a puree. Scrape sides of food processor bowl with a rubber spatula and blend again.
2. Spoon about 1½ tablespoons of the mixture into each segment of an ice cube tray until all the pesto sauce is gone.
3. Freeze overnight, then put the frozen pesto cubes in a zip-lock freezer bag and keep frozen until needed.

4. When you are ready to make the sauce, thaw the cubes in the microwave or in a non-stick frying pan. You can add a tablespoon of fat-free half-and-half for each ice cube to make a creamy pesto sauce. Toss about 3 tablespoons of sauce with each ½ cup of pasta, garnish with the vegetables of your choice, and sprinkle with some fresh Parmesan cheese if desired.

Nutritional Facts (*per ⅛ cup of pesto*): 107 calories, 3 g protein, 1.6 g carbohydrate, 10 g fat (2 g saturated fat, 6.5 g monounsaturated fat, 1.5 g polyunsaturated fat, 0.2 g omega-3 fatty acids, 1.3 g omega-6 fatty acids), 3 mg cholesterol, 0.6 g fiber, 127 mg sodium. Calories from fat: 84 percent.

47 RE vitamin A, 4 mg vitamin C, 1 IU vitamin D, 1.6 IU vitamin E, 0.1 mcg vitamin B_{12}, 10 mcg folate, 65 mg calcium, 1.6 mcg selenium.

Cruciferous Vegetable and Noodle Stir-Fry

This is a different, hearty, and healthful way to use those packages of ramen noodles. By only using one of the seasoning packets, you'll cut down on the sodium.

Makes 4 large servings • Serving size: about 3 cups

2 3-ounce packages chicken or pork ramen noodles and 1 of the seasoning packets
1½ tablespoons canola oil
½ medium cauliflower head (cut away the core and cut the rest into florets)
3 carrots, thinly sliced

2 medium onions, peeled and quartered, then sliced
½ small head cabbage, thinly sliced
2 tablespoons light soy sauce
1 teaspoon sesame oil

1. Cook ramen noodles (without the seasoning packet) in a medium saucepan according to the package directions, then drain well. Add the noodles back to the saucepan; sprinkle the seasoning over the top of noodles and stir to blend; set aside.
2. Heat canola oil in a large, heavy nonstick skillet over medium heat. Add cauliflower,

carrots, and onions. Cover skillet and cook, stirring frequently, until crisp-tender (about 6–8 minutes).

3. Spread cabbage over the top of the vegetables, stir, cover the pan, and continue to cook, stirring frequently, until cabbage is softened (about 3 minutes). Remove from heat. Mix in cooked noodles, soy sauce, and sesame oil, and serve!

Nutritional Facts (*per serving*): 328 calories, 11 g protein, 51 g carbohydrate, 10 g fat (1.5 g saturated fat, 3.8 g monounsaturated fat, 3.6 g polyunsaturated fat, 0.7 g omega-3 fatty acids, 2.9 g omega-6 fatty acids), 0 mg cholesterol, 11.5 g fiber, 916 mg sodium. Calories from fat: 29 percent.

1,131 RE vitamin A, 115 mg vitamin C, 0 IU vitamin D, 4 IU vitamin E, 0 mcg vitamin B_{12}, 159 mcg folate, 156 mg calcium, 9.5 mcg selenium.

Oven-Roasted Red Potatoes and Carrots

These roasted red potatoes and carrots are super-easy to prepare and are loaded with vitamin-rich carbohydrates!

Makes 8 servings • Serving size: about 1¼ cups

1 1-ounce envelope dry onion soup mix
3 tablespoons olive oil
3 tablespoons apple juice

2 pounds red potatoes, cut into eighths
(about 8 cups)
2 cups baby carrots

1. Preheat oven to 450 degrees. Line a jelly-roll pan with foil and coat the foil with canola oil cooking spray.
2. Combine the soup mix, olive oil, and apple juice in very large bowl and stir together with a wire whisk. Toss in the red potatoes and carrots, and coat the vegetables well.
3. Spread potatoes and carrots into prepared pan and bake until potatoes and carrots are tender and potatoes are nicely browned (about 30 minutes)—stirring mixture after 15 minutes.

Nutritional Facts (*per serving*): 205 calories, 4 g protein, 36 g carbohydrate, 5.7 g fat (0.8 g saturated fat, 3.9 g monounsaturated fat, 0.7 g polyunsaturated fat, 0.2 g omega-3 fatty acids, 0.4 g omega-6 fatty acids), 0 mg cholesterol, 5.1 g fiber, 349 mg sodium. Calories from fat: 24 percent.

123 RE vitamin A, 20 mg vitamin C, 0 IU vitamin D, 1.3 IU vitamin E, 0 mcg vitamin B_{12}, 34 mcg folate, 31 mg calcium, 1.7 mcg selenium.

Potatoes with Leeks and Gruyère

This is a super dish for dinner. It can even be baked, cooled, covered, and refrigerated the day before. Simply re-warm, covered, in 350-degree oven for about 25 minutes.

Makes 12 servings • Serving size: about 1 cup

1 tablespoon olive or canola oil

1 pound leeks (white and pale green parts only), thinly sliced

1 8-ounce package of light cream cheese, at room temperature

1 teaspoon salt

1 teaspoon ground black pepper

¼ teaspoon ground nutmeg (or more if desired)

1 cup lowfat milk

1 large egg

½ cup egg substitute

2 pounds frozen shredded hash browns, thawed somewhat

2 cups Gruyère cheese, grated (about 8 ounces)

1 teaspoon dried parsley flakes or Italian herb blend

1. Preheat oven to 350 degrees. Coat a 13x9x2-inch baking dish with canola oil cooking spray.
2. Add olive oil to large nonstick skillet over medium heat. Add leeks and sauté until tender, about 8 minutes. Remove from heat and set aside.
3. Blend cream cheese, salt, pepper, and nutmeg in food processor or mixer. If using a mixer, slowly add milk and eggs one at a time and beat just until blended. If using a food processor, add both the milk and eggs and pulse just until blended. Stir leeks, shredded potatoes, and Gruyère into milk mixture and pour into prepared baking dish. Sprinkle parsley flakes or herbs over the top if desired.
4. Bake dish at 350 degrees until cooked through and top is brown, about 50–60 minutes.
5. Cool slightly and serve.

Nutritional Facts *(per serving)*: 217 calories, 11.5 g protein, 20 g carbohydrate, 10 g fat (6 g saturated fat, 2.9 g monounsaturated fat, 0.5 g polyunsaturated fat, 0.1 g omega-3 fatty acids, 0.4 g omega-6 fatty acids), 48 mg cholesterol, 2 g fiber, 404 mg sodium. Calories from fat: 41 percent.

118 RE vitamin A, 3 mg vitamin C, 15 IU vitamin D, 0.8 IU vitamin E, 0.4 mcg vitamin B_{12}, 20 mcg folate, 243 mg calcium, 4 mcg selenium.

Ranch Beans

Beans are a great high-fiber complement to many main dishes, but this recipe has some meat in it so it actually can serve as the main entrée, too!

Makes 8 large servings • Serving size: about 1½ cups

1 28-ounce can baked beans (I use Maple Cured Bacon Bush's Baked Beans)

1 medium onion, diced

1 medium bell pepper, diced

1 14-ounce package Louis Rich Turkey Polska Kielbasa sausage links or similar less-fat sausage, cut into small, bite-size chunks

½ cup catsup

1 14.5-ounce can diced tomatoes, drained well, if desired

1–2 tablespoons chili powder (use 1 tablespoon for a kid-friendly version)

3 tablespoons Worcestershire sauce

3 tablespoons apple cider or white vinegar

½ cup brown sugar, packed

1 tablespoon minced or chopped garlic (1 teaspoon garlic powder can be substituted)

1 or 2 dashes cayenne pepper (or more to taste)

1 tablespoon red pepper flakes (optional)

1. Add baked beans, onion, pepper, sausage, ketchup, and tomatoes to slow cooker.
2. Sprinkle chili powder, Worcestershire sauce, vinegar, brown sugar, garlic, salt if desired, cayenne, and red pepper flakes if desired, over the top of the bean mixture and stir well.
3. Heat in slow cooker on high for 2–4 hours or on low for 8–10 hours.

Note: This recipe was designed for a slow cooker, but if you want to use a Dutch oven, preheat oven to 350 degrees, add all the ingredients to the Dutch oven, stir, and bake for 1 hour.

Nutritional Facts *(per large serving)*: 296 calories, 14.5 g protein, 50 g carbohydrate, 4.5 g fat (1.3 g saturated fat, 1.5 g monounsaturated fat, 1.3 g polyunsaturated fat, 0.2 g omega-3 fatty acids, 0.2 g omega-6 fatty acids), 32 mg cholesterol, 6 g fiber, 945 mg sodium. Calories from fat: 14 percent.

68 RE vitamin A, 30 mg vitamin C, 0 IU vitamin D, 0.6 IU vitamin E, 0 mcg vitamin B$_{12}$, 13 mcg folate, 140 mg calcium, 0.7mcg selenium.

Rice with Black Beans

A nice stand-alone dinner dish or side dish that will give you not one but two high-carb foods that may help you sleep better at night—rice and beans! *Makes 8 servings*

1 onion, chopped

1 tablespoon canola oil

1 14.5-ounce can Mexican-style stewed
   tomatoes

1 15-ounce can black beans, rinsed and
   drained

½ teaspoon dried oregano

2 teaspoons garlic, minced or chopped

⅔ cup water

1½ cups instant brown rice

Dash hot sauce or Tabasco, or ½ teaspoon
   cayenne pepper (optional)

1. Add oil to a large saucepan over medium heat. Add onion and sauté until tender and just starting to turn golden brown.
2. Add tomatoes, beans, oregano, garlic, and water. Bring to a boil. Stir in brown rice and a dash of hot sauce if desired. Bring mixture back to a boil, then reduce heat to simmer and cover.
3. Simmer mixture for 5 minutes. Turn off heat and let mixture sit in saucepan for 5–10 minutes. Serve!

Nutritional Facts *(per serving):* 146 calories, 5 g protein, 27 g carbohydrate, 2.5 g fat (0.2 g saturated fat, 1.1 g monounsaturated fat, 0.6 g polyunsaturated fat, 0.2 g omega-3 fatty acids, 0.4 g omega-6 fatty acids), 0 mg cholesterol, 4.5 g fiber, 336 mg sodium. Calories from fat: 16 percent.

    28 RE vitamin A, 10 mg vitamin C, 0 IU vitamin D, 1 IU vitamin E, 0 mcg vitamin B_{12}, 11 mcg folate, 43 mg calcium, 0.7 mcg selenium.

5.

Aphrodisiacs for Menopausal Women Only

What's a chapter on aphrodisiacs doing in a cookbook about menopause? There are two main reasons why "stimulating and suggestive" recipes might come in handy for you right about now.

1. One of the symptoms of menopause is vaginal dryness, and one of the most natural ways to improve this symptom is to enjoy sex more often.
2. Decreased libido is a major complaint of postmenopausal women— as our estrogen level decreases, our sexual appetite can decrease along with it. Certainly eating seductively shaped aphrodisiacs can't hurt.

Somewhere between 25 and 63 percent of American women regularly experience some form of sexual dysfunction, with the most prevalent age group being—you guessed it—postmenopausal women. Enter aphrodisiacs. It certainly doesn't hurt to stack the sexual odds in your favor by enjoying foods and dishes that suggest sex to your mind and body. That's what this chapter is all about. Basically, aphrodisiacs aim to stimulate the love senses of sight, smell, taste, and touch with an elite list of erotic ingredients. Do they really work? Can eating certain foods and even the simple act of eating arouse sexual desire? The answer is *yes*—but not in the way you might think.

The bad news is that no food has been scientifically proven to directly or chemically stimulate human sex organs. The good news is that sexual desire can indeed be influenced by food and eating, but in a psychophysiological (the science of the correlation between mind and body) way. In other words, foods and eating can be used to suggest sex to the mind and in turn help stimulate desire in the body.

The Five Historical Types of Aphrodisiacs

Most aphrodisiacs in history fall into the categories of five general hypotheses that somehow survived centuries. Hypotheses are unproven theories—not necessarily fact. They are as follows:

The Temperature Hypothesis

Foods that create warmth and moisture (such as chili or curry) were said to be sexually stimulating or arouse "heated" passion, while cold foods (such as lettuce and melon) were said to "chill" passion.

The Striking-Resemblance Hypothesis

Foods that have the appearance of male or female genitalia are believed to increase desire. The infamous oyster is an example, as are some fruits and root vegetables like carrots.

The Remarkable Reproduction Hypothesis

Reproductive organs and eggs (fish roe and bird eggs, for example) are thought to increase sexual desire and potency.

The Exotic-Erotic Hypothesis

Foods that are considered exotic or rare, and consequently expensive, are believed to be sexually exciting foods. When many of these foods, such as potatoes and cocoa, became more generally available, their sexual-stimulant reputation tended to wane, demonstrating that the fact that these foods and ingredients were exotic, rare, and/or expensive was actually more attractive and sexually powerful for most people than the foods themselves.

The Stimulate-the-Senses Hypothesis

Foods that stimulate the senses in a pleasurable way were thought to stimulate passion.

Examples of Erotic Edibles

Throughout history, vegetables such as onions, turnips, leeks, squash, asparagus, artichokes, and watercress were thought not only to stimulate desire but also to increase sperm count. Shapely fruits like the apple and curvaceous pear were seen by some as erotic edibles. And the heavily seeded fruits like pomegranates and figs were compared to the "seeds of fertility."

And what about those infamous oysters? Alas, oysters, despite the sexual exploits attributed to their powers, are composed entirely of elements that do not and cannot possibly chemically stimulate the genitals of either gender: namely, water, protein, carbohydrate, fat, some salts, glycogen, and negligible quantities of inorganic minerals like potassium and calcium. Apparently, the oyster can thank its shape and mucouslike texture for its aphrodisiac acclaim.

Chocolate is arguably one of America's favorite "comfort foods," but to the ancient Aztecs, chocolate offered a whole lot more than comfort—it was considered to be a powerful aphrodisiac. In the early 1980s, researchers thought they had solved the mystery of America's love affair with chocolate. They detected the amphetamine-like chemical phenylethylamine (PEA) in chocolate. PEA is a central nervous system stimulant, usually present in the human brain, that is thought to help arouse our emotions—a veritable love-drug, so to speak. But the human body actually absorbs very little PEA from chocolate—not enough to play with our emotions, anyway. So it seems the most sexual thing about chocolate is its sensual taste and its smooth and creamy melt-in-your-mouth texture, which, in my opinion, is not too shabby!

Herbs and Other Supplements

There are plenty of herbs and other supplements that claim to decrease vaginal dryness and improve libido in menopausal women, but can they really? The two that researchers have noted as the most promising are vitex and ginseng.

Vitex (Also Called Chasteberry)

This herb contains hormonelike substances and has been recommended for vaginal dryness at menopause and also for enhanced libido. Test-tube and animal studies suggest that vitex may inhibit prolactin, which does suggest a mechanism where it may possibly improve libido. Prolactin is a hormone produced by the pituitary gland, and too much prolactin (a condition called hyperprolactinemia) may be associated with amenorrhea (lack of menstruation) in women and reduced sexual potency in men.

Ginseng

Ginseng is commonly named as an aphrodisiac, but this claim has yet to be substantiated by medical evidence. On the plus side, in Asia ginseng is commonly included in herbal mixtures used for the treatment of sexual dysfunction. And lab and animal studies have shown that Asian and American ginseng may enhance libido and copulatory performance, possibly due to its direct effects on the central nervous system and gonadal tissues. An Italian research paper states that ginseng is thought to promote vitality and appears to be safe when used appropriately. But documented side effects include hypertension, diarrhea, restlessness, breast pain, and vaginal bleeding.

Aphrodisiacs Through the Centuries

Believe it or not, it's not just overworked, stressed-out, contemporary couples who are pursuing foods to boost their sexual appetite. The search for aphrodisiacs started hundreds of years ago.

In medieval times (1000–1600 A.D.), the aphrodisiacs of the period were mainly marine delicacies, such as boiled crab, steamed and boiled clams, and also roasted fowl and their eggs.

During the twelfth century, many written references were made to the sexual powers of wine. One researcher wrote, "It arouses the erection all the more when one enjoys the wine with desire."

The spice trade from Asia added herbs and spices into the aphrodisiac equation in fourteenth-century Europe. Historical accounts suggest that many of the herbs and spices introduced to Europe had sterling aphrodisiac reputations in their native regions. Some of the spices in question were cloves, anise seed, cinnamon, ginger, white pepper, cardamom, and thyme. These spices were probably imported for reasons other than their preserving and flavoring talents.

The fact that both sweet and white potatoes were new to Europe in the sixteenth century and imported for a time helped perpetuate the belief that these foods possessed magical sexual powers. Other vegetables joined the ranks of the potato as aphrodisiacs in the sixteenth to eighteenth centuries, namely carrots, as vegetable or juice and carrot seeds, and asparagus juice.

By the eighteenth century, the influence of phallic-shaped foods, such as eel, carrots, and asparagus, had definitely taken hold. The appearance of food became a vital ingredient in measuring a food's aphrodisiac potential. The Doctrine of Signatures theory, which hypothesized that nature attempts to help mankind by revealing a plant's interior virtues through its external appearance, probably helped this belief along. Various bulb vegetables thought to resemble testicles, like the onion, were thought to affect a man's potency.

Say It with a Whisper

So with all of this suggestiveness, what *can* we as menopausal women use as edible antidotes to sexual apathy or declining sexual appetite? Phallic and shapely foods will probably always be seen as aphrodisiacs, and exotic and rare foods will probably always serve to impress and excite us with their newness and expense. But hopefully today we have grown to appreciate the value of certain foods that suggest sex with subtlety—with a whisper instead of a shout. I'm talking about the difference between serving a dessert that people will glare at and surmise, "That's a penis, all right!" and the more subtle brandy-baked banana, half-drizzled with chocolate sauce.

Other Sensual Food Qualities

Other than drawing on the shape of foods to suggest sex, there are thought to be five other food qualities that elicit sensuality:

- smooth
- rich
- creamy
- exotic
- spicy

Many of the recipes in this chapter draw on these five characteristics.

DOES ALCOHOL HELP OR HURT?

In the late sixteenth century, many scientists documented both the sexually inhibiting and enhancing properties of alcohol. One sixteenth-century researcher wrote that "excessive alcohol is a sexual depressant rather than a stimulant and wine taken moderately does the opposite." They even knew 400 years ago that some amount of alcohol could help our sexual desire, while too much alcohol could hinder it! Recent Italian research noted that "alcohol has a direct toxic effect on the gonads [testes and ovaries] and the liver." But how much is too much? The amount of alcohol that would impede us as drivers seems to also impede us as lovers. This might be more than two drinks a night for men and more than one drink a night for women.

The Nose Always Knows

Certain smells, such as chocolate chip cookies, bread, or an apple pie baking in the oven, can immediately fill our mind with visions of favorite or familiar foods and tantalize our taste buds with anticipation, recalling memories or feelings from some pleasurable past experience associated with that smell. Consider boosting your sexual appetite with smells that stimulate this normally neglected sense. You can surround your soiree environment with pleasant and/or erotic smells. This is a very individual thing. Some might enjoy musk or lavender, for example.

Just Have Fun

Given all that we've just learned about the myths and the truths of aphrodisiacs, have some fun with the following recipes. Some have certain shapes, textures, and ingredients that are thought to arouse your senses. Of course, a lot has to do with your partner and the way you feel about this special person, but hopefully these potentially stimulating recipes will add to your new adventures together.

Suggestive Recipes for Menopausal Women Only

Asparagus Finger Rolls

This is a super-convenient, super-sexy appetizer. You can make the rolls ahead of time and freeze them in a resealable bag, then take them out and bake them right before you need them. *Makes 12 servings • Serving size: 1 long piece*

12 fresh asparagus spears, trimmed
12 slices higher-fiber and higher-calcium
    white bread (IronKids crustless
    works great)

8 ounces light cream cheese
½ cup blue cheese
¼ cup egg substitute

1. Add asparagus spears to a large microwave-safe dish. Add ¼ cup water, cover, and microwave on high until the lower parts of the stalks are barely fork-tender (about 3–4 minutes. Drain immediately and rinse in ice-cold water to stop the cooking process.
2. Remove crusts from the bread and flatten the slices with a rolling pin. Combine cheeses and egg substitute in a mixing bowl and beat with an electric mixer until blended.
3. Spread the cheese and egg substitute mixture evenly over the bread slices. Place an asparagus spear on the edge of each slice and roll the bread up firmly, making sure the tip of the asparagus peeks through the rolled-up bread. Place the rolls side by side in a

resealable bag and chill in the refrigerator for 24 hours, or freeze in a bag until ready to use.

4. Preheat oven to 400 degrees. Take rolls out of the refrigerator or freezer, spray each roll all the way around with canola oil cooking spray, and place them seam-side-down on a cookie sheet.

5. Bake the rolls at 400 degrees until brown (about 10 minutes if from the refrigerator, and 15 minutes if from the freezer). Serve immediately!

Nutritional Facts (*per serving*): 121 calories, 7 g protein, 14 g carbohydrate, 4.3 g fat (2 g saturated fat, 0.8 g monounsaturated fat, 0.5 g polyunsaturated fat, 0.1 g omega-3 fatty acids, 0.4 g omega-6 fatty acids), 11 mg cholesterol, 2 g fiber, 299 mg sodium. Calories from fat: 32 percent.

81 RE vitamin A, 2 mg vitamin C, 4 IU vitamin D, 0.4 IU vitamin E, 24 mcg folate, 72 mg calcium, 9.5 mcg selenium.

Crab Puff Bites

These are really easy to make, and the crab filling puffs up nicely as the bites bake and turn light brown. They are fun to eat with your fingers, and crab is considered an erotic ingredient by many. But you can crank up the aphrodisiac angle on these bites by topping each crab bite with a green olive slice, a pimento, or a caper.

Makes about 24 bites ▪ Serving size: 3 bites

1 8-ounce package reduced-fat crescent-roll dough

1 4-ounce package light cream cheese, softened (about ½ cup)

½ cup fresh crab meat, all shells removed

1 tablespoon fat-free half-and-half

1 tablespoon Parmesan cheese, shredded

¼ cup reduced-fat sharp cheddar cheese, shredded (about 1 ounce)

1 tablespoon green onion, finely chopped (or more to taste)

½ teaspoon Worcestershire sauce

Pinch paprika

1. Preheat oven to 375 degrees. Lightly coat a nonstick mini-muffin pan with canola oil cooking spray.

2. Roll out crescent dough and use a 2-inch biscuit cutter to cut out 24 rounds (don't worry about the perforations in the prepackaged dough). Line each of the mini-muffin cups with the dough, stretching each round out slightly to fit.

3. Add cream cheese, crab meat, half-and-half, Parmesan and cheddar cheese, green onion, and Worcestershire sauce to small mixing bowl and beat on low, scraping sides of bowl often, until mixture is nicely blended.

4. Spoon a heaping teaspoon measure of the filling into each dough-lined mini-muffin cup. Sprinkle paprika over the top of the bites, and add possible garnishes, if desired (green olive slice, a pimento, or a caper).

5. Bake for 15 minutes at 375 degrees, or until puffy and light brown.

Nutritional Facts (*per serving*): 145 calories, 6.5 g protein, 13 g carbohydrate, 7 g fat (2.4 g saturated fat, 0.1 g monounsaturated fat, 0.1 g polyunsaturated fat, 0 g omega-3 fatty acids, 0 g omega-6 fatty acids), 15 mg cholesterol, 0 g fiber, 353 mg sodium. Calories from fat: 43 percent.

51 RE vitamin A, 0.3 mg vitamin C, 2 IU vitamin D, 0.1 IU vitamin E, 4 mcg folate, 58 mg calcium, 3 mcg selenium.

Food-Processor Olive-Cheese Balls

I revamped this holiday favorite using my handy-dandy food processor, and also cut as many food-prep corners as possible. I used an 8-ounce bag of preshredded 2 percent reduced-fat sharp cheddar cheese, which gave me exactly the amount of cheese I needed. I didn't melt the butter or margarine as in the original recipe—I didn't need to now that I was food processing the whole shebang. I did have to increase the milk a tad to help bind the mixture together. No pastry blender needed. No cheese grater. No saucepan. No kneading. Just a food processor, a measuring cup and spoon, and a couple cookie sheets, and you'll be in business.

Makes 34 balls • Serving size: 2 balls

1¼ cups unbleached flour

¼ cup light or fat-free cream cheese

2 cups shredded reduced-fat sharp
    cheddar cheese (an 8-ounce bag
    or preshredded works perfectly)

4 tablespoons butter or margarine (canola
    margarine works fine if the margarine
    contains at least 9 grams of fat per
    tablespoon)

¼ cup lowfat or whole milk

34 pimento- or garlic-stuffed green olives,
    drained well

1. Place flour in food processor. Add cream cheese, cheddar cheese, and butter to food processor bowl. Pulse for about 5 seconds to blend well.
2. Drizzle milk over the top of the mixture and pulse until a dough forms (about 3 seconds). Add another tablespoon of milk if necessary.
3. Wrap a tablespoon of dough around an olive, making sure the top of the olive peeks through the middle. Place the balls about 2 inches apart on a cookie sheet that has been coated with canola oil cooking spray.
4. Cover and refrigerate at least an hour, while preheating oven to 400 degrees. Bake until set, about 15 minutes.

Note: If you don't have the time to let the balls chill in the refrigerator, go ahead and bake them immediately.

Nutritional Facts *(per serving or 2 balls)*: 111 calories, 5 g protein, 8 g carbohydrate, 6 g fat (3.7 g saturated fat, 1.4 g monounsaturated fat, 0.2 g polyunsaturated fat, 0.1 g omega-3 fatty acids, 2 g omega-6 fatty acids), 17 mg cholesterol, 3 g fiber, 306 mg sodium. Calories from fat: 48 percent.

69 RE vitamin A, 1 mg vitamin C, 3 IU vitamin D, 0.4 IU vitamin E, 16 mcg folate, 110 mg calcium, 3 mcg selenium.

Potato Boats

These finger snacks are reminiscent of popular restaurant-style potato skins. You'll make excuses to prepare these again and again. They're a great way to use leftover baked potatoes!

Makes 8 potato boats • Serving size: one boat

4 medium to large russet potatoes, scrubbed, baked, or microwaved, then cooled slightly

about 2 teaspoons canola oil

½ cup reduced-fat cheese, grated (I suggest using part cheddar and part Monterey Jack)

4 strips turkey bacon, fried and crumbled

2 green onions, trimmed and finely chopped

freshly ground pepper

⅓ cup light or reduced-fat ranch dressing for dipping (optional)

1. Preheat oven to 450 degrees. Line a cookie sheet with foil.
2. Cut potatoes in half lengthwise. Scoop out most of the insides with a spoon, leaving about ¼ inch of potato. (You can save the parts you scooped out to make mashed potatoes.)
3. Lightly brush the inside and skin side of the potato halves with canola oil and set them on prepared cookie sheet, skin-side-down. Bake at 450 degrees for about 10 minutes, until light brown.
4. Add cheese, bacon, and green onions to a small bowl and toss together with a fork. Sprinkle the potatoes evenly with the grated cheese mixture. Top with freshly ground pepper if desired.
5. Bake at 450 degrees until cheese is bubbly, about 6 minutes. Serve with ranch dressing for dipping, if desired.

Nutritional Facts: 170 calories, 5 g protein, 23 g carbohydrate, 6.4 g fat (1.7 g saturated fat, 1.2 g monounsaturated fat, 0.7 g polyunsaturated fat, 0.2 g omega-3 fatty acids, 0.5 g omega-6 fatty acids), 14 mg cholesterol, 2.2 g fiber, 259 mg sodium. Calories from fat: 25 percent.

17 RE vitamin A, 12 mg vitamin C, 0 IU vitamin D, 0.4 IU vitamin E, 12 mcg folate, 66 mg calcium, 1 mcg selenium.

Roasted Garlic and Brie Baguette

This is a fun appetizer or light entrée for a couple to share—what with the squeezing of the roasted garlic cloves and the spreading of the melted brie. It's creamy and full of flavor, too. You can use sliced French bread or, if you want to increase some fiber, you can substitute whole-wheat crackers (preferably reduced-fat) or thinly sliced whole-wheat French or sourdough bread. Garnishing each slice with a roasted whole almond or cashew can't hurt the aphrodisiac angle either.

Makes 8 servings • Serving size: 1 large slice or 2 small slices

16 *cloves garlic, still on the bulb*
1 *teaspoon olive oil*
Freshly cracked pepper
Dried oregano leaves
½ *cup brie (without skin)*

16 *thin slices of French baguette (about*
    8 *regular French bread slices)*
16 *whole roasted almonds or cashews*
    (optional)

1. Preheat oven to 350 degrees.
2. Trim the top off the garlic bulb, about ¼ inch, place it on a piece of foil, and drizzle the oil over the top. Sprinkle pepper and oregano over the top of the garlic bulb and wrap it in the foil. Bake about 30–40 minutes.
3. Add brie to small, microwave-safe bowl and cook on high about 1–2 minutes to melt.
4. Squeeze a roasted garlic clove onto a slice of baguette, discarding the garlic skin. Then spread some of the brie on top and garnish one end of the slice with a roasted almond if desired. Repeat with remaining ingredients.

Nutritional Facts (*per serving*): 234 calories, 8 g protein, 35 g carbohydrate, 6.5 g fat (2 g saturated fat, 1.9 g monounsaturated fat, 0.6 g polyunsaturated fat, 0.1 g omega-3 fatty acids, 0.5 g omega-6 fatty acids), 8 mg cholesterol, 2.5 g fiber, 440 mg sodium. Calories from fat: 25 percent.

15 RE vitamin A, 1.3 mg vitamin C, 0.6 IU vitamin D, 1.5 IU vitamin E, 67 mcg folate, 79 mg calcium, 22 mcg selenium.

Smoked Salmon Crostini with Caviar

This recipe is easy to make and yet makes such an elegant appetizer. You can add the caviar garnish if you like, but it really is delicious without it.

Makes 8 appetizer servings • Serving size: 2 slices

16 slices thin, cocktail-size rye bread or sourdough baguette slices

⅔ cup light cream cheese (from a block works best)

1 small bunch scallions, minced (about ½ cup)

1 tablespoon fresh dill, chopped

1 tablespoon capers, chopped

Tabasco sauce

8 ounces thinly sliced smoked salmon, cut into 16 pieces

4 thin slices Bermuda onion, quartered to make 16 wedges

2 teaspoons caviar (optional)

1. Preheat oven to 350 degrees. Place the bread slices on a large nonstick cookie sheet and lightly coat with canola oil cooking spray. Bake until toasted golden, about 8–10 minutes.

2. In a food processor bowl, combine the cream cheese, scallions, dill, capers, and Tabasco. Process until the cheese is fluffy, stopping the machine from time to time to scrape down the sides of the bowl, about 1 minute.

3. Spread the cream cheese mixture onto the toast. Top each slice with a piece of salmon, a wedge of onion, and top each piece with about ⅛ teaspoon of caviar if desired.

Nutritional Facts: 93 calories, 9 g protein, 7 g carbohydrate, 3.3 g fat (1.3 g saturated fat, 0.7 g monounsaturated fat, 0.4 g polyunsaturated fat, 0.2 g omega-3 fatty acids, 0.2 g omega-6 fatty acids), 13 mg cholesterol, 2 g fiber, 730 mg sodium. Calories from fat: 32 percent.

64 RE vitamin A, 1.3 mg vitamin C, 91 IU vitamin D, 0.6 IU vitamin E, 12 mcg folate, 33 mg calcium, 15 mcg selenium.

Chicken Satay Skewers

You can grill the chicken skewers instead of broiling them—either way works great. Just keep in mind that the chicken must be marinated for 8 hours or overnight.

Makes 20 skewers • Serving size: 4 skewers

20 *bamboo or wooden skewers*
4 *boneless, skinless chicken breasts*
¼ *cup lower-sodium soy sauce*
⅛ *cup dark molasses*
⅛ *cup brown sugar, packed*

2 *teaspoons garlic, minced or chopped*
½ *tablespoon no-trans-fat margarine*
   or butter
Juice from ½ large lemon

1. Cover each chicken breast with waxed paper and pound with the flat end of a meat mallet to about ¼ inch thick. Cut each breast into about five long strips.
2. Over medium heat, add soy sauce, molasses, brown sugar and garlic to small saucepan and stir together until the sugar dissolves, about 1–2 minutes. Turn off the heat.
3. Add the margarine and lemon juice, and continue stirring until margarine has melted.
4. Place chicken strips in a shallow dish and pour satay sauce over the top. Cover and let sit in refrigerator for 6–8 hours or overnight.
5. Soak the skewers in water for a few hours or overnight. When ready to cook, thread each strip of chicken onto one of the bamboo skewers and broil on a foil-lined cookie sheet, about 6 inches from the flame, until top is nicely browned, about 2 minutes. Flip skewers and brown other side, about 2 minutes. Serve!

Nutritional Facts (*per serving*): 134 calories, 22 g protein, 6 g carbohydrate, 2 g fat (0.4 g saturated fat, 0.6 g monounsaturated fat, 0.4 g polyunsaturated fat, 0.03 g omega-3 fatty acids, 0.2 g omega-6 fatty acids), 55 mg cholesterol, 0 g fiber, 311 mg sodium. Calories from fat: 13 percent.

11 RE vitamin A, 0.2 mg vitamin C, 11 IU vitamin D, 0.2 IU vitamin E, 4 mcg folate, 33 mg calcium, 17 mcg selenium.

Oysters Rockefeller

In an aphrodisiac chapter, you just know there's going to be a recipe with oysters! This is it—it's rich and delicious and contains almost half the fat of traditional oyster recipes.

Makes 9 servings • Serving size: 2 large or 3 small oysters

1 tablespoon butter or margarine

½ of a 10-ounce package frozen chopped spinach, thawed and drained (but do not squeeze)

¼ cup beer, white wine, or chicken broth

¼ cup onion, minced

1 tablespoon fresh parsley, chopped

1 bay leaf, finely crumbled

¼ teaspoon salt

⅛ teaspoon cayenne pepper or ⅛ teaspoon Tabasco or other hot pepper sauce

½ cup bread crumbs made from fat-free croutons (using the food processor)

18 large or 24 small oysters on the half shell (have the fish counter open them for you, and drain any liquid from the half shell once it is opened)

3 slices less-fat turkey bacon, cooked until crisp, and crumbled

3 tablespoons Parmesan cheese, grated or shredded

Lemon wedges for garnish

1. Preheat oven to 425 degrees. Melt the butter in a 1-quart saucepan over medium heat. Add the spinach, beer, onion, parsley, bay leaf, salt, and cayenne pepper, and cook, stirring occasionally, until the spinach is heated through. Stir in the bread crumbs and remove from the heat.

2. Place the oysters in a baking pan and spoon on the spinach mixture. In a food processor, briefly blend the bacon pieces with the Parmesan cheese. Sprinkle the bacon mixture over the spinach mixture.

3. Bake for 5 to 8 minutes, until lightly brown on top. Garnish with lemon wedges and serve.

Nutritional Facts (*per serving*): 69 calories, 4 g protein, 5 g carbohydrate, 3.5 g fat (1.6 g saturated fat, 1 g monounsaturated fat, 0.7 g polyunsaturated fat, 0.2 g omega-3 fatty acids, 0.4 g omega-6 fatty acids), 24 mg cholesterol, 1 g fiber, 261 mg sodium. Calories from fat: 45 percent.

145 RE vitamin A, 5 mg vitamin C, 91 IU vitamin D, 0.7 IU vitamin E, 28 mcg folate, 61 mg calcium, 20 mcg selenium.

1-2-3 Chocolate Mousse

This popular dessert has three of the five aphrodisiac characteristics; it's smooth, rich, and creamy. Restaurant-quality chocolate mousse can weigh you down because it is soooo rich and dense with calories and fat. With this recipe, we've lightened the mousse, and it's a whole lot easier to whip up than those restaurant recipes. The microwave is used to melt the chocolate; it can also be melted gently in a double boiler.

Makes 6 servings • Serving size: about ⅔ cup

*Any risk of salmonella from using raw eggs is eliminated, because we are using a pasteurized egg substitute made from egg whites, as is the case with Egg Beaters.

1 cup semi-sweet chocolate chips (about 6 ounces)

3 tablespoons egg substitute, at room temperature

1 teaspoon vanilla extract

1 cup prepared French vanilla pudding (you can use instant pudding made with lowfat milk)

2 cups light Cool Whip or light whipping cream

1. Add chocolate chips to a 2-cup glass measure and microwave on low for 2–4 minutes until completely melted when stirred with a spoon. Stir in the egg substitute and vanilla, and set aside to cool for a few minutes.

2. Add prepared pudding and Cool Whip to a medium mixing bowl and stir with spoon. Add in the chocolate mixture, using a plastic scraper to remove it from the measuring cup. Stir until smooth.

3. Spoon the mixture evenly into about 6 small dessert cups and place in refrigerator for about an hour. Enjoy!

Nutritional Facts *(per serving)*: 241 calories, 4 g protein, 33 g carbohydrate, 11 g fat (7.5 g saturated fat, 3 g monounsaturated fat, 0.3 g polyunsaturated fat, 0 g omega-3 fatty acids, 0.3 g omega-6 fatty acids), 3 mg cholesterol, 2 g fiber, 160 mg sodium. Calories from fat: 41 percent.

25 RE vitamin A, 0 mg vitamin C, 44 IU vitamin D, 0.7 IU vitamin E, 5 mcg folate, 58 mg calcium, 1 mcg selenium.

Rum-Glazed Caramelized Banana

It is so easy to make a quick dessert for two with this recipe! Got a banana? You are halfway there. I don't even like bananas, but I love this dessert.

Makes 2 servings • Serving size: ½ of a banana

1 teaspoon butter

1 large banana, halved lengthwise

2 teaspoons brown sugar, packed

2 tablespoons rum, preferably dark

1 tablespoon water

⅛ teaspoon nutmeg, grated

⅛ teaspoon ground cinnamon

2 cookie scoops of light vanilla ice cream (about ¼ cup per scoop)

1 tablespoon toasted mixed nuts, chopped, such as almonds, pecans, macadamia nuts, or peanuts (optional)

1. Melt butter in a 10-inch nonstick skillet over medium heat until foam subsides. Add banana halves, cut-side-down, and shake skillet for 1 minute.
2. Remove skillet from heat and sprinkle brown sugar around the banana. Quickly pour rum around the banana, return the pan to the heat, and continue to cook, shaking skillet occasionally, until sugar begins to melt, about 30 seconds.
3. Reduce heat to low and add water, nutmeg, and cinnamon, and cook until sauce is slightly thickened, about 1 minute.
4. Carefully lift each banana half from pan and place on a dessert plate. Garnish one end of the banana half with a cookie scoop of light vanilla ice cream; drizzle half the sauce over the length of each banana piece and sprinkle nuts over the ice cream if desired.

Nutritional Facts *(per serving)*: 135 calories, 1 g protein, 22 g carbohydrate, 2.2 g fat (1.3 g saturated fat, 0.6 g monounsaturated fat, 0.2 g polyunsaturated fat, 0.1 g omega-3 fatty acids, 0.1 g omega-6 fatty acids), 5 mg cholesterol, 2 g fiber, 22 mg sodium. Calories from fat: 15 percent.

24 RE vitamin A, 7 mg vitamin C, 1.3 IU vitamin D, 0.4 IU vitamin E, 15 mcg folate, 9 mg calcium, 1 mcg selenium.

6.

I'm Not Moody–
I'm This Cranky All the Time!

Do you feel as though you are turning into a menopausal maniac? What is going on? First of all, if you are noticing your mood subtly (or not-so-subtly) shifting lately from elated to irritable or from delighted to depressed, you are not alone. Fluctuating hormones, mainly due to the declining levels of estrogen during perimenopause and after menopause, may be one major cause of menopause-related mood swings. Of course, not sleeping well night after night and dealing with hot flashes every hour on the hour probably isn't helping matters, either. Here are four possible reasons why some menopausal women become much more moody.

1. Lack of sleep
2. Anxiety about lack of sleep and other symptoms
3. Life changes, such as, children leaving home or caring for aging parents
4 Fluctuating hormones (declining estrogen levels) may be one cause of mood swings.

Improve Your Mood by Destressing Your Day

Working or living under a large amount of stress can mess with your mood—menopause or no menopause. So women who are pre- and postmenopausal and want to improve their mood should definitely try to destress their days and nights. More easily said than done, I know. The following are three ways that stress impacts the way we eat, according to the September 2002 *Food & Fitness Advisor.*

1. The more stressed people are, the more calories they tend to eat.
2. Women who are under stress eat fewer fruits and vegetables than those who aren't stressed.

3. Men who are under stress eat more fatty foods than those who aren't stressed. (And its possible that women react to stress similarly.)

Mood Food

As women, even before menopause, we sometimes feel we are slaves to our hormones. Some of us find ourselves, despite our best intentions, trading in our Dr. Jekyll for Mr. Hyde a few days every month. We call it PMS. Well, many women in the midst of menopause consider PMS to be the little leagues of hormone-induced irritability compared to perimenopause.

What can you eat to keep bad moods few and far between, and good moods plentiful during this hormonally challenging time of your life? That's the million-dollar question—and your husband and family may be willing to pay a million dollars for the answer! Can it really be that simple? There is a lot for the scientific community to learn about how diet influences our moods; we don't have the whole story yet, but we certainly have some clues that could be pointing us in the right direction.

Desperate times call for desperate measures. Recent studies have shown that there are quite a few things we can do food-wise to help stabilize our moods. I advise trying to incorporate as many of the following food suggestions as possible. They also happen to offer many other health benefits to your body in general, so you have nothing to lose in the health department—they are great things to do in and of themselves.

THE FOOD AND MOOD CONNECTION

Basically, the science of food's ability to elevate or deflate our mood is based on this equation:

Dietary changes ⟶ (bring about) ⟶ changes in our brain structure, chemistry and physiology ⟶ (which leads to) ⟶ altered animal behavior!

Three Things You Can Start Doing Today to Elevate Your Mood

One group of researchers recommends that women try three things to improve their moods. I'm warning you right now, two of these are super-easy, but the third is one of the toughest things I've ever had to do.

1. *Work more omega-3 fatty acids (from fish, and also plant sources such as flax) into your day.* Researchers have noted that omega-3 polyunsaturated fatty acids may be mood stabilizers, playing a role in mental well-being.
2. *Eat a balanced breakfast.* Eat lots of fiber and nutrients, and some lean protein and good fats, and whole-grain carbohydrates every single morning. Eating breakfast regularly leads to improved mood, according to some researchers, along with better memory, more energy throughout the day, and feelings of calmness.
3. *If you are overweight, lose weight slowly but surely.* Some researchers advise that slow weight reduction in overweight women can help elevate their mood. Fad dieting isn't the answer, though, because depriving yourself of too many calories and carbohydrates can help instigate irritability. *(Med J Aust 2000 Nov.6; 173 Suppl: S104–5})* I suggest focusing on eating and exercising for the health benefits, and letting the pounds fall where they may. You can find out more about keeping excess weight off in Chapter 8.

Foods That Boost Serotonin Levels

There is some evidence that estrogen may help prevent mood swings by stimulating the production of serotonin—the neurotransmitter that I fondly refer to as the "feel-good" neurotransmitter. Serotonin communicates "happy" messages to your brain, and the more serotonin circulating in your bloodstream, the better your mood will be. Quick, pass the serotonin, please! In contrast, low levels of serotonin can put us in a bad mood and increase aggression, according to some studies. Are there food or nutrients that can actually elevate the level of serotonin in the bloodstream and brain? Of course! The following food components may influence our brain levels of serotonin.

Tryptophan

Tryptophan is a nonessential amino acid. As more tryptophan enters the brain, more serotonin is synthesized in the brain, and our mood improves. Will eating high-tryptophan foods improve your mood? Although tryptophan is found in almost all protein-rich foods, other amino acids are better at passing from the bloodstream into the brain, which is why eating carbohydrates seems to help tryptophan cross the blood/brain barrier.

Folic Acid (folate)

A lack of folic acid in the diet can cause lower levels of serotonin in the brain and bad moods. Some studies suggest that taking folate supplements (there is a day's supply in most balanced multivitamins) and emphasizing folate-rich fruits and vegetables may be helpful for people who are depressed.

When it comes to raising serotonin levels, there is one type of nutrition component that is almost always mentioned: carbohydrates. It is common knowledge to mood experts that carbohydrate consumption increases serotonin release and that protein intake doesn't. We need carbohydrates, and it behooves us to choose our carbohydrates wisely (stressing carbohydrate foods that come with lots of nutrients and fiber, such as whole grains, beans, fruits, and vegetables. This can be a double-edged sword for carbohydrates, though, because many of us may have developed a tendency to overconsume carbohydrates in an effort to make ourselves feel better emotionally.

Dr. Judith Wurtman, a researcher with the MIT Department of Brain and Cognitive Sciences and Clinical Research Center, and a national expert on the issue of food and mood, suspects that many women learn to overeat carbohydrates (particularly snack foods, such as chips or pastries), which are rich in carbs and fats, to make themselves feel better. Using (or abusing) certain foods as if they are recreational drugs is probably a major cause of weight gain for some susceptible women.

I personally feel that it may not be the carbs women are craving in some of these foods, but the combination of carbs and fat. Just think about some of the high-carbohydrate foods we crave, such as potato chips, french fries, chocolate, and ice cream—these foods get most of their calories from fat, not carbohydrates!

So what's the answer to the big carb question? Go for the carbs, but make smart carb choices and balance your smart carbs with a little lean protein and healthier fats. Don't choose products made with refined flours and processed grains, and don't choose foods made with lots of sugar and sweeteners. A little is fine, but a lot can be trouble. There is a whole world of nutrient-rich carbohydrates out there for you to explore. Take a fresh look at whole-grain breads, oats, barley, and brown rice, and all sorts of beans, fruits, and vegetables. When you start going for the carbs with fiber and nutritional value, you will automatically start walking away from those high-fat, high-carb foods women tend to overeat.

Carbs Have a Calming Effect

Thick-crust pizza (if the crust is bready and not greasy), here we come! According to Dr. Judith Wurtman, eating more calories or carbohydrates could end up helping people concentrate to a certain degree by calming them down. That extra crust in the deep-dish pizza may help your body make more serotonin, the feel-good brain chemical that calms you. That's right, all you low-carb dieters out there may be barking up the wrong tree where menopause is concerned!

The results from one Dutch study suggest that when high-stress-prone people eat carbohydrate-rich/low-protein meals, they tend to increase the levels of tryptophan in their brains, and when exposed to stress, these participants did not show a rise in depression or a decline in vigor.

Yet Another Reason to Avoid Alcohol

We know that alcohol consumption, particularly when it is excessive, doesn't encourage quality sleep. That's reason #1 for menopausal women to pass up that second or third glass of wine. We know that alcoholic beverages are full of calories that our bodies can't easily use for energy and therefore are generally converted to fat storage. That's reason #2 for women to be cautious with alcohol. Here's reason #3: there is some scientific evidence pointing to a relationship among serotonin dysfunction, negative mood states, and excessive consumption of alcohol. It's safe to say that alcohol is not a mood stabilizer, and it is probably best for menopausal women to avoid alcohol (particularly when consumed in more-than-moderate quantities) in the interest of discouraging low moods during this hormonally challenging time.

Calling All Chocoholics!

Chocolate and I go way back. I crave chocolate in the middle of the day, almost every day. I'm happy with a chocolate kiss or a handful of trail mix with chocolate chips—I have a little, and I don't feel guilty about it. I feel like it is a chemical thing with me. There aren't many foods I can say I crave on a regular basis, but I do crave chocolate. Some chocoholics say it lifts their spirits.

But what do the experts say? Chocolate may not be a mood lifter for some women. One study in England found that when people who describe themselves as "chocolate addicts" got their chocolate "fix," so to speak, their moods did not improve. The researchers believe that chocolate is clearly a very pleasurable food, but for people who consider their chocolate intake to be "excessive," any pleasure experience is short lived due to the subsequent feelings of guilt.

Selenium: A Mineral the Brain Counts On

It's a strong antioxidant that works with and can replace vitamin E activity, protects polyunsaturated fats, red blood cells, and cell membranes, and is needed for the synthesis of thyroid hormones. One important nutrient that does all that! It's the mineral selenium. The daily recommended intake is about 55 mcg/day for women age 19 and older. But you don't want to overdo selenium, because it is a mineral, which means the body can't get rid of excess amounts. Doses two to three times the recommended daily amounts appear to be harmless, but know that the potential for toxic doses of selenium arise more from selenium supplements than from selenium in food.

So what does this have to do with mood? Five studies have reported an association between low selenium intake and poorer moods. Although the underlying mechanism is unclear, researchers do have some clues. The way the brain metabolizes selenium differs from the way other organs metabolize it; in times of deficiency, the brain retains selenium to a greater extent, leading some researchers to believe that selenium plays an important function in the brain.

It's hard to be in a good mood when you are tired. So I thought it might be helpful to run through some tips on high-energy eating—how to fight fatigue with food.

Tip #1:   Your body needs fuel for energy, so give it a well-balanced, healthy diet and drink plenty of water.

Tip #2:   Start your day with a lower-fat, higher-fiber breakfast.

Tip #3:   Eat small amounts of food more frequently during the day, when possible, instead of eating about two large meals. (Large meals zap you of your energy, and so does going hungry when you have large gaps between meals.)

Tip #4:   Include fresh fruits and vegetables, whole grains, lean meats (or vegetable proteins if you are a vegetarian), and lowfat dairy in your diet to make sure your diet is balanced and you are getting all the nutrients you need.

Tip #5:   Don't fill up on high-fat or sugary foods. They tend to leave you feeling sluggish—if not right away, then shortly thereafter.

10 Recipes to Boost Your Mood

Our best plan of attack to boost our moods through food choices is to enjoy fish more often, to choose carbohydrates that contain fiber and important nutrients, and to make a point of adding folic acid and selenium-rich foods to our daily diet. The recipes in this chapter will focus on adding fish, folic acid, and selenium.

Manhattan Clam Chowder

I wanted to include a clam recipe, because clams are one of the top selenium food sources, and they have a bit of omega-3s as well. I took the recipe one step further by adding green soybeans, which will contribute some folic acid. You may be skeptical about adding them, but the texture of the soybeans is actually great in this soup. This is a really easy and tasty recipe, and it takes only about 15 minutes to prepare!

Makes 6 servings • Serving size: about 1½ cups

3 6.5-ounce cans minced clams

2 16-ounce cans diced tomatoes

1 cup onion, chopped

2 large potatoes,
    peeled and chopped

½ cup carrots, finely chopped

1½ cups shelled green soybeans
    (edamame), found in the frozen
    vegetable section of some supermarkets

1 teaspoon salt (optional)

Ground black pepper to taste

½ teaspoon dried thyme

1. Drain clams and reserve liquid. Add enough water to reserved liquid to make 3 cups of stock.
2. In a large saucepan, pour clam juice and water mixture, tomatoes, onion, potatoes, carrots, soybeans, salt, pepper, and thyme. Bring the mixture to a gentle boil; then cover and simmer for 30–35 minutes.
3. Remove the pan from the heat. Mash the vegetables slightly to thicken the broth. Add the clams to the saucepan and continue to simmer until thoroughly hot, about 8–10 minutes. Serve hot.

Nutritional Facts *(per serving)*: 225 calories, 12 g protein, 39 g carbohydrate, 3.1 g fat (0.4 g saturated fat, 0.6 g monounsaturated fat, 1.4 g polyunsaturated fat, 0.2 g omega-3 fatty acids, 1.2 g omega-6 fatty acids), 7 mg cholesterol, 5.6 g fiber, 780 mg sodium. Calories from fat: 12 percent.

351 RE vitamin A, 38 mg vitamin C, 0 IU vitamin D, 0.2 IU vitamin E, 0 mcg vitamin B_{12}, 68 mcg folate, 160 mg calcium, 1.5 mcg selenium.

Cranberry-Pecan Chicken Salad

This salad is served on a bed of romaine lettuce—the romaine lettuce is rich in folic acid, while the chicken is a top selenium source. Don't skip the last step of letting it chill in the refrigerator for at least an hour—this gives all the different flavors more time to blend and intensify. This recipe is a great way to use leftover chicken from a barbecue.

Makes 4 salads • Serving size: about 3 cups

2 cups cooked chicken breast, cubed, firmly packed

½ cup dried cranberries (you can substitute dried chopped cherries)

½ cup celery, finely chopped

2 green onions, chopped

¼ cup green or yellow bell pepper, finely chopped

½ cup pecans, toasted and coarsely chopped (toast pecans by baking in 300-degree toaster oven until lightly browned, about 4 minutes)

4 teaspoons mayonnaise (light mayonnaise can be substituted)

6–8 tablespoons fat-free or light sour cream

½ teaspoon paprika

½ teaspoon seasoning salt (optional)

Ground black pepper to taste

8 cups romaine lettuce, freshly washed, drained, and chopped

1. Place chicken, cranberries, celery, onions, pepper, and pecans in a medium bowl and toss together.
2. Add mayonnaise, sour cream, paprika, and seasoning salt to a 1-cup measure or small bowl and stir until well blended.
3. Pour mayonnaise mixture over chicken mixture and stir together until everything is well coated. Add black pepper to taste. Chill in the refrigerator for at least 1 hour. Serve over romaine lettuce.

Nutritional Facts *(per serving)*: 285 calories, 16.5 g protein, 19.5 g carbohydrate, 16 g fat (2 g saturated fat, 7.7 g monounsaturated fat, 5.6 g polyunsaturated fat, 1.2 g omega-3 fatty acids, 3.4 g omega-6 fatty acids), 41 mg cholesterol, 3 g fiber, 89 mg sodium. Calories from fat: 50 percent.

73 RE vitamin A, 8 mg vitamin C, 5 IU vitamin D, 1.3 IU vitamin E, 0.3 mcg vitamin B_{12}, 23 mcg folate, 65 mg calcium, 13 mcg selenium.

Quick-Fix Chicken Caesar Salad

This will hopefully become a favorite light dinner for those hot summer nights—I know it is in my house. The chicken gives it a dose of selenium, while the romaine lettuce contributes folic acid.

Makes 4 servings • Serving size: about 2½–3 cups

OIL-FREE CROUTONS:

4 slices sourdough bread (or 8 slices baguette) cut into ¾-inch cubes

1 tablespoon Parmesan cheese, shredded

½ teaspoon garlic powder

¼ teaspoon freshly ground pepper

DRESSING:

¼ cup regular bottled Caesar salad dressing that uses canola oil or olive oil

¼ cup sparkling apple cider or regular apple juice

SALAD:

8 cups Caesar-style salad greens (either prepackaged salad or from one large head of romaine lettuce, inner leaves only), torn into bite-size pieces

3 tablespoons Parmesan cheese, shredded

2 boneless and skinless chicken breasts, broiled or barbecued and cut into ½-inch strips

1. To make croutons, preheat oven to 325 degrees. Place the bread cubes in a single layer on a cookie sheet. Spray the top of the bread with canola oil cooking spray. Flip the bread and spray again. In a small cup, blend 1 tablespoon Parmesan cheese with garlic powder and pepper, and sprinkle evenly over the bread cubes. Bake until the croutons are golden brown and crisp all the way through, about 5–10 minutes. Let cool.

2. In a small bowl, whisk the Caesar salad dressing with the apple cider; set aside.

3. Place the lettuce in a large serving bowl and top with the croutons, 3 tablespoons of Parmesan cheese, then the chicken breast strips. Drizzle the dressing over the top and gently toss to blend well. Serve!

Note: If you want to broil your chicken breasts, preheat the broiler, then spray both sides of each chicken breast with canola or olive oil cooking spray. Lightly sprinkle both sides of chicken with

1–2 teaspoons of Mrs. Dash Lemon Pepper, or a similar salt-free seasoning blend. Broil each side for about 4–6 minutes, or until chicken is golden brown and cooked throughout. Let cool, then slice into ½-inch strips.

Nutritional Facts *(per serving including croutons)*: 337 calories, 23 g protein, 42 g carbohydrate, 8.3 g fat (1.9 g saturated fat, 1.5 g monounsaturated fat, 1 g polyunsaturated fat, 0.2 g omega-3 fatty acids, 0.8 g omega-6 fatty acids), 46 mg cholesterol, 4 g fiber, 659 mg sodium. Calories from fat: 22 percent.

300 RE vitamin A, 28 mg vitamin C, 7.5 IU vitamin D, 2 IU vitamin E, 0.2 mcg vitamin B_{12}, 209 mcg folate, 140 mg calcium, 37 mcg selenium.

Simple Salmon Pasta Salad

This upscale pasta salad features the nutritionally sought-after salmon, a rich source of omega-3 fatty acids and selenium. Adult servings can be given a sprinkle of capers, which will set off the flavors of the salmon and dill nicely. The pasta is a top source of folic acid and selenium.

Makes 4 servings • Serving size: 2 cups

2½ cups dried bow-tie or rotelle pasta (whole-grain pasta can be used)

1 cup salmon, (broiled, smoked, or grilled and flaked, all bones removed)

1 cup asparagus pieces, lightly steamed or micro-cooked but still tender (another vegetable can be substituted)

3 green onions, finely chopped (optional)

1 tablespoon capers (optional)

DRESSING:

1 tablespoon mayonnaise (light mayonnaise can be substituted)

3 tablespoons fat-free sour cream (light sour cream can also be used)

1 tablespoon lemon juice

1½ teaspoons Dijon mustard

½ teaspoon dried dillweed (or 2 teaspoons fresh dill)

Black pepper to taste

1. Boil water in a large pot and begin cooking pasta. Continue to boil until the pasta is cooked al dente (about 8 minutes), and rinse and drain well. (While pasta is cooking, you can microwave the asparagus and broil the salmon if you haven't already done so.)

2. Combine the cooked pasta, salmon, asparagus, and onions if desired in large serving bowl; toss to blend.

3. Combine dressing ingredients in a small bowl and whisk or stir until smooth. Pour dressing over pasta salad and stir to mix. Add more black pepper to taste and a sprinkling of capers if desired.

4. Chill in the refrigerator until ready to serve.

Nutritional Facts (*per serving*): 252 calories, 15 g protein, 29 g carbohydrate, 8.5 g fat (1.9 g saturated fat, 3 g monounsaturated fat, 3 g polyunsaturated fat, 0.7 g omega-3 fatty acids, 0.1 g omega-6 fatty acids), 32 mg cholesterol, 2 g fiber (whole-grain pasta will be add about 3 to 4 grams of fiber per serving), 164 mg sodium. Calories from fat: 30 percent.

85 RE vitamin A, 6 mg vitamin C, 0 IU vitamin D, 1.3 IU vitamin E, 1.1 mcg vitamin B_{12}, 99 mcg folate, 46 mg calcium, 17 mcg selenium.

Spinach Salad with Brazil Nuts and Gorgonzola

Prewashed bags of spinach greens make this recipe a cinch to prepare! This lightened salad looks and tastes so wonderful with its fresh spinach (a rich source of folic acid), crumbled bacon and gorgonzola cheese, toasted Brazil nuts (which are rich in selenium) and garlic-herb dressing. I actually took this salad to a friend's house for a little dinner party—it's that type of salad! *Makes 6 servings • Serving size: about 2½ cups*

8–9 ounce package fresh spinach, thoroughly washed and dried (about 12 cups)

3 slices Louis Rich turkey bacon, cooked carefully until crisp and crumbled

¼ cup Gorgonzola cheese, crumbled

⅓ cup Brazil nuts, coarsely chopped (and toasted if desired)

DRESSING:

2 tablespoons extra-virgin olive oil or canola oil

2 tablespoons honey

¼ cup fat-free sour cream

¼ cup rice vinegar or white wine vinegar

3 tablespoons fresh basil, chopped (or 1 teaspoon dried)

2 cloves garlic, minced (about 1½ teaspoons)

Salt and freshly ground pepper to taste

Note: If you can't buy Brazil nuts separately, buy a can of mixed nuts and pick out the Brazil nuts—they are the really large nuts that look like oversized garlic cloves. To toast the nuts, bake on a cookie sheet at 350 degrees in the middle of the oven or toaster oven until lightly brown, about 5 minutes.

1. Remove tough stems from spinach; tear the large leaves into bite-size pieces.
2. Just before serving, place spinach greens in a salad bowl. Sprinkle bacon pieces, Gorgonzola, and nuts over the top.
3. In small bowl (a small food processor also works well), whisk together the olive oil, honey, sour cream, vinegar, basil, garlic, and salt and pepper until smooth and creamy. Pour over the spinach mixture and toss. Serve immediately!

Nutritional Facts *(per serving)*: 197 calories, 6 g protein, 11 g carbohydrate, 15 g fat (5.3 g saturated fat, 4.1 g monounsaturated fat, 0.8 g polyunsaturated fat, 0.1 g omega-3 fatty acids, 0.7 g omega-6 fatty acids), 11 mg cholesterol, 2 g fiber, 196 mg sodium. Calories from fat: 68 percent.

287 RE vitamin A, 12 mg vitamin C, 0 IU vitamin D, 2 IU vitamin E, 0 mcg vitamin B_{12}, 74 mcg folate, 85 mg calcium, 0.6 mcg selenium.

Baked Italian Salmon

This is a great recipe for beginner cooks! The salmon is our omega-3 contributor, and if you serve it with brown rice or white or whole-wheat pasta, you'll get a dose of selenium, too. Add a side of vegetables—such as okra, broccoli, spinach, asparagus, or brussels sprouts—and you'll get some folic acid as well. Any extra sauce that collects in the foil pouch with the salmon can be poured over your vegetables or rice.

Makes 2-3 servings • Serving size: about 4 ounces salmon

2 cloves garlic, minced or chopped	¼ teaspoon salt
1 tablespoon extra-virgin olive oil	¼ teaspoon ground black pepper
2 tablespoons white wine (flavored vinegar can be substituted)	1 tablespoon lemon juice
	1 tablespoon fresh parsley, chopped
1 teaspoon dried basil	3 4-ounce salmon fillets

1. In a medium glass bowl, prepare marinade by mixing garlic, olive oil, wine, basil, salt, pepper, lemon juice, and parsley.
2. Place salmon fillets in a medium glass baking dish and cover with the marinade. Marinate in the refrigerator about 1 hour, turning occasionally.
3. Preheat oven to 375 degrees. Place both fillets on a large sheet of aluminum foil, cover with marinade, and wrap foil around them, sealing well. Place the foil packet in the glass dish, and bake 35 to 45 minutes, until easily flaked with a fork. Serve!

Nutritional Facts (*per serving if 3 servings per recipe*): 236 calories, 26 g protein, 1.2 g carbohydrate, 12.5 g fat (1.9 g saturated fat, 6.3 g monounsaturated fat, 3.7 g polyunsaturated fat, 2.3 g omega-3 fatty acids, 0.9 g omega-6 fatty acids), 71 mg cholesterol, 0.1 g fiber, 251 mg sodium. Calories from fat: 47 percent.

20 RE vitamin A, 5 mg vitamin C, 283 IU vitamin D, 3 IU vitamin E, 3.1 mcg vitamin B_{12}, 32 mcg folate, 22 mg calcium, 48 mcg selenium.

Cashew Chicken Salad Sandwich

This is a delicious lunch or dinner sandwich that uses quite a few ingredients that are high in selenium, but we keep it lower in fat by using fat-free sour cream and just a hint of mayonnaise. Serving it on some fresh whole-grain bread will give the fiber and nutrient totals a boost. A serving also contains at least 30 percent of the U.S. recommended daily amount of all the B vitamins, 35 percent of the RDA of folic acid, 17 percent of the RDA calcium, 53 percent of the RDA magnesium, and 122 percent of the RDA of selenium.

Makes 2 large sandwiches • Serving size: 1 sandwich

2 cups skinless roasted chicken breast, chopped (from a rotisserie chicken you can buy at your local grocery store)

⅓ cup celery, finely chopped

2 green onions, finely chopped (optional)

¼ cup cashew pieces

2 teaspoons mayonnaise (light mayonnaise can be substituted)

¼–⅓ cup fat-free or light sour cream

¼ teaspoon curry powder

¼ teaspoon chicken broth powder (optional)

SERVING SUGGESTIONS:

fresh whole-grain or whole-wheat bread

lettuce leaves

tomato slices

1. Place chicken, celery, onion (if desired), and cashew pieces in a medium bowl and toss well.

2. In small bowl, blend mayonnaise, sour cream, curry, and chicken broth powder (if desired) together, drizzle over chicken mixture, and blend well.

3. Serve chicken salad on the bread of your choice, topped generously with lettuce leaves and tomato slices.

Nutritional Facts *(per serving with whole wheat bread, lettuce and tomato)*: 462 calories, 38 g protein, 40 g carbohydrate, 16.5 g fat (3.8 g saturated fat, 7.7 g monounsaturated fat, 4.7 g polyunsaturated fat, 0.2 g omega-3 fatty acids, 2.4 g omega-6 fatty acids), 78 mg cholesterol, 6 g fiber, 435 mg sodium. Calories from fat: 32 percent.

123 RE vitamin A, 15 mg vitamin C, 15 IU vitamin D, 2 IU vitamin E, 0.4 mcg vitamin B_{12}, 90 mcg folate, 143 mg calcium, 47 mcg selenium.

Crab Quesadillas

Fresh cilantro adds a nice touch, but if you don't have any, try using one of the new cilantro-flavored bottled salsas. This recipe's feature ingredient, crab, is high in selenium and folic acid, and contains omega-3 fatty acids. Each flour tortilla adds about 17 mcg of selenium.

Makes 4 quesadillas • Serving size: 1 quesadilla

¾ teaspoon garlic, minced

¼ cup green onion, chopped

1 jalapeño pepper, stemmed, seeded, and finely diced (or chop 1 mild bottled jalapeño or a canned fire-roasted chili, Ortega brand)

½ pound crabmeat, washed, drained well, and shredded into bite-size pieces

2 teaspoons mayonnaise (light mayo can be substituted)

2 tablespoons fat-free sour cream

Salt to taste

4 teaspoons minced fresh cilantro

4 lowfat flour tortillas

2–3 ounces (½ heaping cup) reduced-fat Monterey Jack cheese, shredded

Salsa, fat-free or light sour cream, and avocado (optional)

1. Add garlic, green onion, jalapeño, crabmeat, mayonnaise, sour cream, salt, and cilantro to a medium-size mixing bowl; blend well.

2. Place 1 tortilla on a microwave-safe plate and sprinkle a heaping ⅛-cup measure (or 2 tablespoons) of the cheese over the top of the tortilla.

3. Spoon ⅓ cup of crab mixture evenly over half of the tortilla.

4. Microwave on high for 2–3 minutes or until cheese is melted. Remove from microwave and fold the half without the crab over to make a quesadilla.

5. Repeat the above steps with remaining tortillas, cheese, and crab mixture.

6. If desired, brown and crisp quesadillas by heating in a nonstick frying pan over medium heat for 1 minute per side. Serve each quesadilla immediately with salsa, sour cream, and/or avocado if desired.

Nutritional Facts *(per serving)*: 246 calories, 19 g protein, 25 g carbohydrate, 8 g fat (3 g saturated fat, 0.7 g monounsaturated fat, 1.4 g polyunsaturated fat, 0.3 g omega-3 fatty acids, 0.1 g omega-6 fatty acids), 71 mg cholesterol, 2 g fiber, 608 mg sodium. Calories from fat: 29 percent.

70 RE vitamin A, 5 mg vitamin C, 2.3 IU vitamin D, 0.9 IU vitamin E, 4.3 mcg vitamin B_{12}, 31 mcg folate, 257 mg calcium, 23 mcg selenium.

Salmon Dijon

This is a wonderful way to prepare fresh salmon fillets in the oven. Salmon is bursting with omega-3 fatty acids, so I wanted to give you a few salmon recipe options in this chapter. The canola oil will contribute some plant-derived omega-3s too. Even though this recipe has a few high-flavor ingredients, they work together well—none of them are overpowering.

Makes 4 servings • Serving size: 4 ounces salmon

2 teaspoons canola oil

2 tablespoons fat-free half-and-half

3 tablespoons Dijon mustard

1½ tablespoons honey

¼ cup dry bread crumbs

¼ cup pecans, walnuts, or pine nuts,
   finely chopped by hand or in a small
   food processor

4 teaspoons chopped fresh parsley
   (or 2 teaspoons dry flakes)

4 4-ounce fillets salmon,
   skin removed

Salt and pepper to taste (optional)

1 lemon, for garnish

1. Preheat oven to 400 degrees. Line a 9x13-inch baking pan with foil. Coat the foil with canola oil cooking spray.
2. In a small bowl or small food processor, mix together canola oil, fat-free half-and-half, mustard, and honey. Set aside.
3. In another bowl, mix together bread crumbs, pecans, and parsley.
4. Dip each salmon piece first in the mustard mixture and then in the bread-crumb mixture, coating well. Place salmon on prepared pan. Coat top of fillets lightly with canola oil cooking spray.
5. Bake salmon 12 to 15 minutes, or until it flakes easily with a fork in its thickest section.
6. Season with salt and pepper, if desired, and garnish each piece with a wedge of lemon.

Nutritional Facts (*per serving*): 308 calories, 29 g protein, 12 g carbohydrate, 15.5 g fat (2 g saturated fat, 7.6 g monounsaturated fat, 5.9 g polyunsaturated fat, 2.5 g omega-3 fatty acids, 2.6 g omega-6 fatty acids), 72 mg cholesterol, 1 g fiber, 351 mg sodium. Calories from fat: 45 percent.

30 RE vitamin A, 2 mg vitamin C, 289 IU vitamin D, 3.1 IU vitamin E, 3.1 mcg vitamin B_{12}, 36 mcg folate, 65 mg calcium, 49 mcg selenium.

Microwave Salmon in Berry Sauce
with Lemon Rice

This is a beautifully colored and flavored dish. You might be skeptical about cooking the whole dish in the microwave, but it really works well.

Makes 4 servings • Serving size: about 2 cups

1½ cups brown Basmati rice, unrinsed
    and uncooked (white can be
    substituted, but brown is a top
    selenium source)

2¾ cups chicken broth (low-sodium may be
    used), subtract ½ cup broth if using
    white rice

2–3 tablespoons lemon juice

⅔ cup frozen petite green peas

Salt and pepper to taste

4 4-ounce center-cut salmon fillets (about
    1½-inch thick at thickest part), skin
    and bones removed

¼ cup bottled light raspberry vinaigrette
    (Newman's Own makes a light
    raspberry-walnut dressing that
    tastes terrific)

1 tablespoon fresh parsley, finely chopped
    (or 1 teaspoon dry flakes)

Freshly ground black pepper to taste

1. Place rice, broth, and lemon juice in a 2-quart microwave-safe dish and cook on high, uncovered, about 25 minutes (steam holes should appear in rice).

2. Sprinkle peas over the rice, cover dish, and cook on high about 5 more minutes (until rice is fully cooked and peas are lightly cooked). Add salt and pepper to taste if desired. Set covered dish aside while you make the salmon.

3. Coat an 8- or 9-inch round or square microwave-safe, covered casserole dish with canola oil cooking spray. Place the salmon pieces in the dish, folding the thin sides under if necessary so that the fillets are of even thickness. Drizzle the raspberry vinaigrette over the salmon and sprinkle parsley and pepper over the top.

4. Cover (or use microwave-safe plastic wrap to cover dish) and microwave on high for 6 minutes. If your microwave does not have a turntable, turn the casserole a quarter turn every 2 minutes so the fish cooks evenly.

5. Take the dish out of the microwave and let it stand a few minutes (without uncovering). Test the salmon in the thickest part with a fork. If it isn't cooked throughout,

microwave on high for another minute or two until done. Serve each salmon fillet on a mound of rice and spoon the berry sauce (the sauce left in the bottom of the salmon dish) over the top if desired.

Nutritional Facts *(per serving)*: 492 calories, 35 g protein, 64 g carbohydrate, 11.5 g fat (2.3 g saturated fat, 3.6 g monounsaturated fat, 4.2 g polyunsaturated fat, 2.3 g omega-3 fatty acids, 0.6 g omega-6 fatty acids), 74 mg cholesterol, 4.5 g fiber, 354 mg sodium. Calories from fat: 21 percent.

31 RE vitamin A, 10 mg vitamin C, 283 IU vitamin D, 2 IU vitamin E, 3.1 mcg vitamin B_{12}, 43 mcg folate, 36 mg calcium, 48 mcg selenium.

7

What Was I Saying?
I Must Be Having One of Those
Menopause Moments

Have you been losing your train of thought mid-sentence? Or have you ever paraded into a room but once you got there you couldn't remember what you were going there to get? Welcome to my world.

With aging comes cognitive decline. But we don't have to take this lying down. Researchers are also trying to figure out ways we can slow or offset this natural aging process. There is much more to learn, but we already have some great clues to help us preserve brain function. And the good news is that these are simple things we can do.

Foods That Boost Brain Power

Can you get back the mental alertness you feel you have lost? Some experts believe your diet—what you eat and how much—can play a big role in your mental abilities as you age. Here are some foods to choose to help boost your brain function.

Get Fruity!

Eating blueberries will slow your brain from aging. Well, it isn't quite that simple, but more and more research is showing that the phytochemical family polyphenolics (specifically, the anthocyanins, of which blueberries, cranberries, and boysenberries are good sources) may help prevent the brain from aging. Polyphenolic phytochemicals may help the brain by enhancing the signals of brain cells, and possibly the rate at which they are created. Decreasing that rate is associated with greater rates of cognitive decline.

One study found that supplementing rats' diets with extracts from blueberries, cranberries, black currants, or boysenberries improved some aspects of their learning and memory, and the blueberry and cranberry diets also improved motor performance in the rats.

And Don't Forget Your Veggies

Population studies have consistently shown that a fruit- and vegetable-rich diet is associated with the reduced risk of many age-related diseases, such as cancer, heart disease, stroke, dementia (especially Alzheimer's), and some of the functional declines associated with aging. Many researchers feel these anti-aging benefits come from the effects of the antioxidants and phytochemicals in the whole fruit or vegetable, and that you wouldn't get the same effects if you just fed people a single antioxidant or phytochemical. So if you think you can get the antioxidants you need by popping a chewable vitamin-C tablet instead of eating your broccoli, give that idea up. You need to consume the fruits and vegetables as nature made them.

Antioxidants and Aging

Oxidative damage (when cells in your body combine with oxygen in such a way that they become damaged) may be linked to increased rates of aging. Eating ample antioxidant-rich foods should slow the rate of aging. A large study in Switzerland discovered that people in their 60s who had the highest blood levels of vitamin C and beta-carotene—in almost all cases from food, not supplements—scored higher on memory tests than those with relatively low levels.

Some recent studies on aging and canines indicated that a diet rich in antioxidants (including fruits and vegetables) actually slowed—but did not reverse—formation of fatty deposits in the arteries. The researchers think a high-antioxidant diet may promote successful brain aging in humans, too.

The two antioxidants that have been linked to better memory and reasoning ability are vitamin C and beta-carotene. Where do you find them? In fruits and vegetables! Look to the yellow-orange and dark green veggies for beta-carotene, and dark green veggies and citrus fruits for vitamin C.

Are There Any Other Brain-Worthy Vitamins?

Luckily, there are two additional brain-worthy vitamins that we should definitely mention: folic acid (folate) and vitamin B_{12}—both of which are easy to incorporate in a healthy diet. Here's how they influence brain function.

A group of Scottish and British researchers believe that these two vitamins may be the key to controlling levels of homocysteine, a natural chemical compound linked not only to memory loss but also heart disease.

Here's where the vitamins come into play. When B_{12} and folic acid are in good supply in your body, they seem to protect against problems caused by homocysteine. And it looks like the early bird catches the worm, too. The earlier you correct deficiencies of B_{12} and folic acid, the better off you will be. Dr. Barry Reisberg, professor of psychiatry at the NYU School of Medicine, believes that although correcting this nutrient deficiency might not help retrieve lost memory, it can help save you from further losses. In his study, men and women between the ages of 63 and 78 who had higher blood levels of B_{12} and folic acid scored higher on four of six cognitive tests, including tests on memory. For a list of our best food sources of folic acid and B_{12}, see the Appendix.

Yet Another Reason to Eat Soy

Remember the polyphenols (phytochemicals found in fruit) that you read about at the beginning of this chapter? Well, soy is one of the richest food sources of isoflavones, which are phytochemicals in the polyphenols family. Soy consumption has been linked to a lowered incidence of diseases associated with aging such as artherosclerosis, cancer, osteoporosis, and cognitive decline.

Researchers also think isoflavones may help our brain function and play an important role in the prevention of aging. How? Isoflavones may work together with other antioxidants and they may convert to stronger antioxidants in the body too. So far we have some animal studies and three short-term human trials that suggest that soy foods and isoflavones may improve several aspects of cognition and memory, particularly in postmenopausal women, but some scientists believe the preliminary data on soy's cognitive benefits look encouraging.

Tyrosine: Another Brainpower Booster?

Tyrosine is a nonessential amino acid, which means our body can make it from the components of the essential amino acids. So if it is not essential, why would eating tyrosine-rich foods help us during and beyond menopause? It all comes down to the two brain chemicals: epinephrine and dopamine.

Epinephrine and dopamine govern mental alertness. Both are made by the body from tyrosine. When you're engaged in sustained mental activity, you need to replace the tyrosine in your body; you'll find it in some high-protein foods. You don't need a large amount of these high-protein foods, either—2 to 3 ounces will do just fine. Researchers in the Netherlands discovered that tyrosine (consumed in a protein-rich drink) improved cognitive performance and reduced blood pressure in cadets who were participating in a demanding military combat-training course.

Smart Fats for the Brain

Low levels of omega-3 fatty acids may be linked to Alzheimer's, because the first lipid change in the disease is a decreased level of DHA (one of the long-chain omega-3s that we get from fish), which is needed for various enzyme systems involved in signaling mechanisms in the brain. DHA is actually present in the nerve endings in our brain. We get DHA from fish (the fattier the fish, the better—such as salmon and sardines), but our bodies also convert 5 percent of the plant omega-3s we consume to DHA. Some of the best plant sources of omega-3s are ground flaxseeds, canola oil, cauliflower, broccoli, and red kidney beans.

Analysis of data from the renowned Framingham Heart Study also found that low plasma DHA levels, associated with low fish intake, were also associated with an increased risk of Alzheimer's Disease and all-cause dementia (defined as the deterioration of mental state with absence or reduction of intellectual faculties).

Balanced Blood Sugars

Type 2 diabetes runs in my family, so I get a little nervous every time I get blood or urine tests. I'm counting on the fact that if I exercise regularly, avoid obesity as I age, and continue to enjoy a healthful diet, I am likely not to inherit type 2 diabetes. Well, now I have another reason to keep following my plan. A new study has discovered that when your blood sugar levels rise to abnormal levels, you're not only starting to walk down the diabetes road, but your memory may suffer and your brain may actually shrink as well.

The lead author of the study, Dr. Antonio Convit, Medical Director for the Center for Brain Health at the New York University School of Medicine, reminds all of us that if you exercise regularly and eat well, generally you will have healthier blood sugar levels.

The people most at risk for memory issues due to abnormal blood sugars are people with diabetes and people who are considered prediabetic (that is, people with impaired glucose tolerance). This group of prediabetic adults is no small number, either—about 16 million people in the United States between the ages of forty and seventy-four have prediabetes, according to the National Institute of Diabetic, Digestive, and Kidney Disease website.

In the study, Convit and his colleagues evaluated thirty adults, ages fifty-three to eighty-nine; none were diabetic but some had higher than normal blood sugar levels. Those with the lowest scores on the mental tests had the poorest glucose tolerance. The part of the brain responsible for learning and recent memory (the hippocampus) was actually physically smaller in that group. The researchers suggest that the hippocampus may become damaged and begin to atrophy because it isn't able to absorb enough glucose for fuel.

This study demonstrates an association (but not necessarily cause and effect) between poor glucose tolerance and memory problems. Researchers have known for years that diabetics have more memory problems than nondiabetic people their own age. I personally saw the mental decline in my father as he got older, after years and years of out-of-control high blood sugar levels. So this adds yet another reason to avoid obesity, stay fit, and eat a healthy diet.

Tell Me What to Eat to Help Prevent Alzheimer's Disease

Alzheimer's disease is a devastating and debilitating neurodegenerative condition, and the most common cause of dementia among the elderly. Now that we are approaching menopause, it behooves us to try and reduce the risk of as many diseases associated with aging as possible. The disease related to the loss of mental ability is Alzheimer's. You've probably known someone who has suffered from it. It goes without saying that we don't want it, so how do we stop it?

We still know very little about the primary causes of Alzheimer's disease, and it remains incurable today. But the following is what we have learned about helping to prevent Alzheimer's through the foods we choose:

- **Eat your fruits and vegetables, and make sure your multivitamin provides folate and a daily dose of the other B vitamins as well.**

   There is the possibility that low levels of folic acid or high levels of homocysteine in the blood might promote the breaking down of the neurons in the nervous system. But there is something we can do about it. Blood homocysteine levels can be safely lowered by eating foods and taking supplements containing folic acid and other B vitamins.

- **Eat fish two to three times a week.**

- **Would you like some green tea with that?**

   There is a strong possibility (based on test tube and mice studies) that the polyphenols in green tea may significantly delay the progression of neurodegenerative disorders such as Alzheimer's disease.

- **Lowfat eating = low Alzheimer's risk?**

   We don't know for sure, but results from recent studies done at the Department of Neurology at Case Western University in Cleveland, Ohio, raise the possibility that a lowfat (less than 36 percent of calories from fat), high-antioxidant diet protects against Alzheimer's.

What You Drink and How Much May Be Part of the Problem

Not only does what you are eating help or hurt your memory, but so does what and how much you are drinking—of alcohol, that is. Research shows that heavy drinkers have more problems with daily memory tasks, such as remembering to return a phone call or send a birthday card, compared to people who drink very little.

A recent study also found that even moderate levels of drinking have an impact on cognitive function. People who drink 10 to 24 glasses of wine per week, for example, performed significantly worse in long-term memory tests than participants who drank little or no alcohol.

"Alcohol consumption has a significant effect on memory," concludes the study's author Jonathan Ling, Ph.D. "A typical heavy user of alcohol is likely to report 31.16 percent more problems with long-term aspects of prospective memory than someone who does not drink."

Join the Coffee Klatch Crew

I know many people think coffee makes them more alert but are they really? Actually, coffee may help you as you age. Coffee has been shown to improve reaction time, says Judith Wurtman, Ph.D., director of the women's health program at the MIT Clinical Research center in Boston. But she warns not to overdo it—drink too much coffee and you may be too scattered to concentrate on the task at hand.

Lower Your Blood Pressure for Your Heart *and* Your Brain

There is some evidence that high blood pressure may lead to lower mental function. A recent National Institute on Aging study adds more fuel to this fire. In the study, people in their mid-fifties and older with high blood pressure experienced more brain atrophy and scored lower on language and memory tests than others of the same age with normal blood pressure.

So that means that heeding advice to keep your blood pressure down is not only good for your heart but your brain as well. The most recent food guidelines for this comes from a very successful diet and hypertension study called the DASH (Dietary Approaches to Stop Hypertension) eating plan. The study found that blood pressure was lowered with an eating plan that was low in saturated fat, cholesterol, and total fat but higher in fruits (4–5 servings a day), vegetables (4–5 servings a day), and lowfat or fat-free dairy foods (2–3 servings a day). The diet also included whole-grain foods, fish, poultry, and nuts while reducing red meat, sweets, and sugary beverages. The following are a few exciting things you should know about the DASH eating plan and the study.

- The results were dramatic, especially for people in the study with high blood pressure.
- The blood pressure reductions came fast—within two weeks of starting the plan.
- Keep in mind that while each diet step lowers blood pressure, the combination of following the eating plan and reducing your intake of sodium gives the biggest bang for your buck and may help prevent the development of high blood pressure.

Ginkgo Is Probably Not
the Herbal Answer

Old Chinese texts say that ginkgo has the power to benefit the brain, among other things. The Memory Clinic in Bennington, Vermont, says there is not enough research to indicate that ginkgo is safe and effective as a memory booster. The clinic just completed a randomized, double-blind, placebo-controlled trial on the dose of ginkgo recommended on herbal packaging for improving memory. They were particularly interested in testing ginkgo's abilities, because they find that 25 percent of their memory-clinic patients are taking ginkgo or related supplements. The trial showed that when elderly people take ginkgo following the manufacturer's recommendation, it has no effect on learning, memory, or related cognitive function.

Healthy Eating Tips for
Mind Maintenance

So what specific things can we do, diet-wise, to maintain our brain in as peak condition as possible?

- To increase your mental alertness, eating enough food and energy is important. But you don't want to go overboard and eat "too much," because that will quickly turn you from a mental stallion to a sleepy slug, as more blood from your general circulation rushes to your digestive tract and less goes to your brain, making you slower and more sluggish.
- Balance quality carbohydrates with some protein in all your meals. Not only will the protein-rich foods help replenish some of the tyrosine that is important to the brain, but they are also thought to improve cognitive function after the breakfast meal, possibly by encouraging a more moderate glucose metabolism.
- If you are looking to boost mental power in the morning, it's a good idea to include these breakfast-friendly protein-containing foods:

lowfat cottage cheese	peanut butter
lowfat yogurt	whole-grain toast
scrambled eggs or omelets (you can make them with half egg substitute and half high-omega-3 eggs if you desire)	higher-fiber hot or cold cereal, as long as you eat them with some protein

- To avoid a mid-afternoon slump, try adding these protein-rich foods to your lunch:

Chicken	Fat-free or lean lunch meats
Turkey	Hard-boiled eggs (or eggs cooked
Veggie burgers	any way without fat), plain or
Lean burgers	with fat-free mayo

Some lunch no-nos are french fries and sugary caffeinated sodas (one soda can contain 16 teaspoons of sugar). While the caffeine in a cola may provide a momentary blast of mental alertness, the sugar will let you down hard and fast.

- Keep some of the carbs! Carbohydrates can help calm you and help you resist distractions.
- Eat a diet rich in fruits, vegetables, and whole grains.
- Diets rich in vitamin E and other antioxidants (particularly vitamins A and C) may help counter damage to brain cells and may aid your memory.
- Are you trying to keep your mental alertness and eat high-fat meals, too? If you eat a lot of fat and try to be quick on your feet and with your mind, you'll find that you just can't. Studies show that diets high in fat cause fatigue. And fatigue doesn't help your mind stay quick.
- Take a good, hard look at your alcohol consumption. If you are a moderate to heavy drinker (drinking two or more alcoholic drinks a day), your memory and brain function could benefit from cutting way back.
- Keep in mind that as we age, we lose some of our ability to absorb nutrients from the food we eat. So it becomes especially important to make wise food choices and to take a "just in case" vitamin/mineral supplement (such as Centrum Silver).
- A nighttime note: If you plan amorous activities, cut out the fried food and heavy sauces at dinner, Dr. Judith Wurtman (MIT researcher and expert on the aging brain) says. "If not, you will go from perky to pathetic—that is, fried or rich, high-fat foods can turn you from alert to sleepy and sluggish."

Recipes to Feed Your Brain and Memory During Menopause

Brimming with Blueberry Muffins

These muffins are super-moist and full of blueberries with a crispy cinnamon crumb topping. My picky daughter even loved these muffins! If you don't want to use soy flour, just add ¾ cup of whole-wheat flour instead of ½ cup.   *Makes 9 muffins • Serving size: one muffin*

½ cup whole-wheat flour
¼ cup whole soy flour
¾ cup white flour
½ cup white sugar
½ teaspoon salt
2 teaspoons baking powder
3 tablespoons canola oil
1 large egg
*½ cup plus 2 tablespoons fat-free
    half-and-half*
1¼ cups fresh or frozen blueberries

TOPPING:
⅓ cup white sugar
⅓ cup white flour
1½ teaspoons ground cinnamon
*2 tablespoons no-trans- or low-trans-fat
    margarine (for example, Land O'
    Lakes Fresh Buttery Taste Spread or
    Smart Balance)*
2 teaspoons fat-free half-and-half

1. Preheat oven to 400 degrees. Line muffin pan with muffin liners.
2. Add flours, sugar, salt, and baking powder to large mixing bowl and beat on low to combine.
3. Add canola oil, egg, and 9 tablespoons of fat-free half-and-half to dry mixture, and beat on low just until combined.
4. Fold in blueberries. Fill muffin cups until pretty full (using ¼ cup measure).
5. To make crumb topping: Place sugar, flour, and cinnamon in a small food processor bowl and pulse briefly to blend. Add margarine and 1 teaspoon fat-free half-and-half and pulse briefly until a crumb mixture forms. Add 1 more teaspoon half-and-half if

crumb mixture isn't quite moist enough. (If you don't have a small food processor, blend the sugar, flour and cinnamon mixture together with a fork. Then cut in the margarine and half-and-half with a fork until a moist crumb mixture forms.)

6. Sprinkle crumb topping evenly over the muffins (about 1 tablespoon of crumb mixture per muffin) and bake for 20–25 minutes, or until done. Serve.

Nutritional Facts: 256 calories, 5 g protein, 40 g carbohydrate, 8.5 g fat (1 g saturated fat, 4 g monounsaturated fat, 2.3 g polyunsaturated fat, 0.5 g omega-3 fatty acids, 1.2 g omega-6 fatty acids), 24 mg cholesterol, 2.2 g fiber, 269 mg sodium. Calories from fat: 30 percent.

45 RE vitamin A, 1 mg vitamin C, 16 IU vitamin D, 2 IU vitamin E, 0.1 mcg vitamin B_{12}, 30 mcg folate, 112 mg calcium, 12 mcg selenium.

Cream of Mango Soup

Mango is high in beta-carotene and vitamin C, and is a good source of folic acid. This chilled mango soup will also help cool you down and give your calcium totals a boost, too. You can add a sprinkle of blueberries or sliced strawberries as a colorful garnish.

Makes 3 servings • Serving size: about 1 cup

2 mangos, peeled, seeded, and cubed   *1 lemon, zested and juiced*
(about 2 cups)   *1½ cups fat-free half-and-half*
2–3 tablespoons sugar to taste

1. Place mango cubes, sugar, lemon juice, lemon zest, and juice and half-and-half in a blender or food processor.
2. Blend just until smooth and creamy.
3. Garnish with blueberries or strawberries if desired, and serve chilled.

Nutritional Facts *(per serving)*: 206 calories, 10.5 g protein, 42 g carbohydrate, 0.6 g fat (0.2 g saturated fat, 0.2 g monounsaturated fat, 0.1 g polyunsaturated fat, 0.04 g omega-3 fatty acids, 0.02 g omega-6 fatty acids), 5 mg cholesterol, 2 g fiber, 150 mg sodium. Calories from fat: 3 percent.

578 RE vitamin A, 37 mg vitamin C, 102 IU vitamin D, 2 IU vitamin E, 0.3 mcg vitamin B_{12}, 28 mcg folate, 383 mg calcium, 0.4 mcg selenium.

Homestyle Lentil Soup

The wonderful cold weather side dish or entrée contains one of the top folic acid–rich ingredients (lentils) as well as foods high in several of the nutrients mentioned in this chapter (beta-carotene, vitamin C). This recipe also works well for the chapter on moodiness. Not only is it rich in folic acid, if you serve it with a couple of slices of whole-wheat bread, you'll get a daily dose of selenium as well. *Makes 8 servings • Serving size: about 1½ cups*

3 medium onions, diced

4 fresh garlic cloves, minced (about 2 teaspoons)

3 tablespoons olive oil

8 cups chicken broth (use low-sodium broth if desired)

1 pound dried lentils, washed and picked over

2 potatoes, washed and diced

4 Roma tomatoes, quartered

2 large carrots, diced

2 tablespoons fresh oregano leaves, finely chopped (or 1½ teaspoons dried oregano leaves)

¾ teaspoon freshly ground black pepper

Salt to taste

1. In a large pot, sauté the onion and garlic in olive oil until lightly browned.
2. Add all other ingredients and bring to a boil.
3. Cover and let soup boil for 15 minutes.
4. Lower heat to a simmer and cook 1 hour. Serve.

Nutritional Facts (*per serving*): 339 calories, 20 g protein, 51 g carbohydrate, 7.0 g fat (1.6 g saturated fat, 4.2 g monounsaturated fat, 0.9 g polyunsaturated fat, 0.1 g omega-3 fatty acids, 0.7 g omega-6 fatty acids), 4 mg cholesterol, 15 g fiber, 119 mg sodium. Calories from fat: 20 percent.

77 RE vitamin A, 17 mg vitamin C, 0 IU vitamin D, 1.6 IU vitamin E, 0 mcg vitamin B_{12} 314 mcg folate, 66 mg calcium, 5.5 mcg selenium.

Mango or Papaya Chicken Salad

I love to make this satisfying salad in the summer for a cool, light dinner, using leftover grilled chicken from the day before. The broccoli is rich in folic acid, beta-carotene, and vitamin C, the mango contributes vitamin C and beta-carotene, and the chicken gives you a bit of vitamin B_{12}. If you want to substitute some rinsed and drained black beans for the broccoli, be my guest. The black beans will also boost your folate intake for the day.

Makes 2 large entrée salad servings or 4 smaller salads • Serving size: 1 small salad

2 boneless, skinless chicken breasts, roasted or barbecued

1 cup papaya or mango, cut fruit into bite-size pieces

½ large avocado, pitted and peeled, cut into bite-size pieces

⅛ cup green onions, finely chopped

1 cup broccoli florets, lightly steamed and chopped (rinsed and drained black beans can be substituted)

½ cup chopped vine-ripened tomatoes (any type) or cherry tomatoes, halved

DRESSING:

1 tablespoon mayonnaise

3 tablespoons fat-free sour cream (light can also be used)

2 tablespoons orange juice

1–2 teaspoons orange zest, finely chopped (optional)

Freshly ground pepper to taste

¼ cup roasted and lightly salted nuts or soynuts

1 cup chopped tomato

1. Cut the cooled chicken into bite-size pieces. Combine chicken, papaya or mango, and avocado in medium serving bowl. Stir in onions and broccoli.
2. In a small bowl, blend the dressing ingredients well. Drizzle half the dressing over the salad ingredients and toss to blend. Chill until served. Garnish each serving with ¼ cup of chopped tomato and a tablespoon or two of soynuts. Serve with the extra dressing on the side.

Note: *Most people prefer the taste of real mayonnaise, so I use only a little in this recipe. If you like light or fat-free mayonnaise, go ahead and use it! It's completely up to you.*

Nutritional Facts *(per small serving)*: 248 calories, 27 g protein, 12.5 g carbohydrate, 10.5 g fat (2 g saturated fat, 4.1 g monounsaturated fat, 2.7 g polyunsaturated fat, 0.1 g omega-3 fatty acids, 0.9 g omega-6 fatty acids), 62 mg cholesterol, 4 g fiber, 94 mg sodium. Calories from fat: 37 percent.

122 RE vitamin A, 51 mg vitamin C, 8.5 IU vitamin D, 2 IU vitamin E, 0.3 mcg vitamin B_{12} 50 mcg folate, 65 mg calcium, 0.2 mcg selenium.

Crab and Shrimp Salad

The crab contributes B_{12} and folic acid, the shrimp give the B_{12} a boost, and the romaine lettuce adds some folic acid and beta-carotene.

Makes 3 servings • Serving size: about 3 cups

1 tablespoon real mayonnaise	½ cup celery, chopped
6 tablespoons fat-free or light sour cream	¼ teaspoon freshly ground pepper (or more to taste)
Juice from ½ lemon	
¼ teaspoon **Old Bay Seasoning** (add more to taste)	2 tablespoons black olives, sliced
	1–2 green onions (white and part of green), chopped
⅓ pound (about 1 cup) shredded cooked crabmeat (imitation crabmeat can be used in a pinch)	6 cups romaine lettuce, rinsed, well drained, and chopped
1 cup bay shrimp (about ⅓ pound)	

1. Combine mayonnaise, sour cream, lemon juice, and Old Bay Seasoning well with a whisk.
2. Stir in crab, shrimp, celery, pepper, olives, and green onion. Chill at least 1 hour.
3. Serve each serving of salad on a bed of chopped romaine lettuce.

Nutritional Facts *(per serving)*: 191 calories, 22 g protein, 12 g carbohydrate, 5.8 g fat (0.9 g saturated fat, 1.7 g monounsaturated fat, 2.5 g polyunsaturated fat, 0.2 g omega-3 fatty acids, 0.5 g omega-6 fatty acids), 134 mg cholesterol, 3 g fiber, 99 mg sodium. Calories from fat: 28 percent.

388 RE vitamin A, 39 mg vitamin C, 0 IU vitamin D, 3.3 IU vitamin E, 3.7 mcg vitamin B_{12}, 192 mcg folate, 170 mg calcium, 38 mcg selenium.

Strawberry Spinach Salad

with Super-Quick Raspberry-Poppy Seed Dressing

This is one of those "toss and go" 3-minute salads. The trick is blending some bottled raspberry salad dressing with some orange juice and poppy seeds. I realize this might be considered cheating, but this is a really easy way to make a dressing with half the fat using good-tasting store-bought salad dressing.

Makes 6 servings • Serving size: about 1½ cups

1 10-ounce bag of pre-washed spinach
   leaves
2 cups strawberries, halved
⅓ cup bottled raspberry salad dressing
⅓ cup orange juice

1 tablespoon poppy seeds
¼ cup sliced almonds, toasted
1 cup orange fruit to garnish perimeter of
   salad serving bowl, such as orange
   segments, peach slices, or mango slices

1. Add spinach leaves and strawberries to a big salad bowl.
2. In a 2-cup measure, blend raspberry salad dressing, orange juice, and poppy seeds together well.
3. Drizzle dressing mixture over the top of salad in bowl and gently toss to blend all ingredients. Sprinkle toasted almonds over the top. Garnish the perimeter of the salad bowl with orange fruit if desired.

Nutritional Facts *(per serving)*: 91 calories, 4 g protein, 12 g carbohydrate, 4 g fat (0.3 g saturated fat, 2 g monounsaturated fat, 1.3 g polyunsaturated fat, 0.5 g omega-3 fatty acids, 0.8 g omega-6 fatty acids), 0 mg cholesterol, 4 g fiber, 259 mg sodium. Calories from fat: 39 percent.

328 RE vitamin A, 65 mg vitamin C, 0 IU vitamin D, 4 IU vitamin E, 0 mcg vitamin B$_{12}$ 117 mcg folate, 101 mg calcium, 1.1 mcg selenium.

Wasabi Creamed Salmon

This recipe calls for 1 tablespoon of real mayonnaise (the original recipe called for ½ cup!), but you can use fat-free or lowfat mayonnaise if you like. The idea of this recipe is to make a creamy, spicy teriyaki sauce to spread over the fillet, topping it with sliced green pepper and onion, and bake it in a foil pouch in the oven or on the grill. If you can't find or don't like wasabi paste, sprinkle in some red pepper flakes instead.

Makes 4 servings • Serving size: about 5 ounces

1 tablespoon mayonnaise (light mayonnaise can be substituted)
⅓ cup fat-free or light sour cream
¼ cup light teriyaki sauce (bottled)
¼ teaspoon wasabi paste (substitute red pepper flakes if you prefer)

1½ pounds salmon fillet, cut into 4 equal-size pieces
Salt and pepper to taste
1 large green bell pepper, seeded and sliced
1 onion, finely chopped

1. Preheat an outdoor grill for high heat or an oven to 400 degrees.
2. In a small bowl, blend mayonnaise, sour cream, teriyaki sauce, and wasabi paste.
3. Lay 4 pieces of foil on a flat surface. Place a piece of salmon on each piece of foil, skin-side-down. Spread teriyaki mixture over each piece of salmon. Season with salt and pepper.
4. Evenly sprinkle green pepper slices and chopped onion over each salmon fillet. Wrap each fillet well with foil, forming each into a self-contained packet. Place on baking sheet if using the oven and cook or grill about 15 minutes or until salmon is easily flaked with a fork at thickest part of the fillet. Serve.

Note: Wasabi powder is available in very small cans in the Asian foods section of some supermarkets. This recipe calls for wasabi paste, which you get by adding some water to the wasabi powder until it forms a paste.

Nutritional Facts *(per serving)*: 318 calories, 35 g protein, 12 g carbohydrate, 13 g fat (2.2 g saturated fat, 4.2 g monounsaturated fat, 5.7 g polyunsaturated fat, 2.8 g omega-3 fatty acids, 0.8 g omega-6 fatty acids), 94 mg cholesterol, 1.5 g fiber, 540 mg sodium. Calories from fat: 38 percent.

73 RE vitamin A, 30 mg vitamin C, 357 IU vitamin D, 3 IU vitamin E, 4 mcg vitamin B$_{12}$ 51 mcg folate, 61 mg calcium, 60 mcg selenium.

Blueberry Blast Smoothie/Shake

This is a fun, refreshing way to work a serving of soy and phytochemical-rich blueberries into your day. I keep a bag of blueberries in the freezer just so I can make this smoothie!

Makes 1 serving • Serving size: about 2 cups

½ cup light or lowfat ice cream or frozen yogurt

⅔ cup frozen blueberries

¼ cup lowfat blueberry yogurt (or other berry-flavored yogurt)

¼ cup vanilla soymilk (lowfat milk can also be used)

1 tablespoon ground flaxseeds

1. Add all ingredients to small food processor or blender and pulse until blended and mixture is smooth.
2. Pour into a serving cup and enjoy with a spoon or straw!

Nutritional Facts *(per serving)*: 281 calories, 10 g protein, 46 g carbohydrate, 7.5 g fat (2.2 g saturated fat, 1.5 g monounsaturated fat, 2.7 g polyunsaturated fat, 1.7 g omega-3 fatty acids, 1 g omega-6 fatty acids), 14 mg cholesterol, 6 g fiber, 104 mg sodium. Calories from fat: 24 percent.

36 RE vitamin A, 4 mg vitamin C, 3 IU vitamin D, 2.2 IU vitamin E, 0.7 mcg vitamin B$_{12}$, 36 mcg folate, 240 mg calcium, 5 mcg selenium.

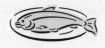

Mango-Boysenberry Crisp

I wanted to add some dessert recipes in this chapter, and a crisp is a nice way to enjoy high-beta-carotene, high-vitamin-C mangos, along with boysenberries, which are rich in phytochemicals that may boost brain power along with an extra dose of vitamin C.

Makes 6 servings

CRISP TOPPING:

⅓ cup walnuts

⅔ cup unbleached white flour

¼ cup ground flaxseeds

3 tablespoons brown sugar

½ teaspoon ground cinnamon

Pinch of salt (if using unsalted butter)

3 tablespoons butter or no- or low-trans-fat canola margarine, melted in microwave

3 tablespoons light pancake syrup (or maple syrup)

FILLING:

2 cups mango, coarsely chopped into a ½ dice

2 cups fresh or frozen boysenberries

¼ cup sugar

3 tablespoons flour

1. Preheat oven to 375 degrees. Toast the walnuts by spreading them in a pie plate and heating in the oven until fragrant, about 7 minutes. Chop the nuts medium-fine and set aside.

2. Combine the flour, flaxseeds, brown sugar, cinnamon, and salt (if using unsalted butter) in a mixing bowl. Drizzle the melted butter and syrup over the top and blend on low speed until crumbly. Add the chopped nuts and mix well. The topping can be prepared a few days ahead of time and refrigerated.

3. Add the mango, boysenberries, and sugar to a large bowl, stir well, and taste. Add more sugar if absolutely necessary. Sprinkle flour over the fruit and mix gently. Spread the mixture into a 2-quart baking dish (a 9x9-inch pan will also work).

4. Spoon the topping over the fruit mixture, pressing down lightly. Place the dish on a baking sheet to catch any overflow. Bake in the center of the oven at 375 degrees until topping is golden brown and the juices are thickened, about 40–45 minutes. Serve warm or cold!

Nutritional Facts (*per serving*): 315 calories, 5.5 g protein, 50 g carbohydrate, 12 g fat (4 g saturated fat, 0.3 g monounsaturated fat, 4.2 g polyunsaturated fat, 1.4 g omega-3 fatty acids, 2.8 g omega-6 fatty acids), 15 mg cholesterol, 6 g fiber, 75 mg sodium. Calories from fat: 34 percent.

276 RE vitamin A, 26 mg vitamin C, 4 IU vitamin D, 2.3 IU vitamin E, 0.01 mcg vitamin B_{12}, 71 mcg folate, 46 mg calcium, 0.8 mcg selenium.

Mango Tart with Blueberries

This may seem like an odd combination of ingredients, but it is a refreshing and delicious dessert boasting two brain-boosting fruits: mangoes and blueberries.

Makes 8 servings • Serving size: 1 slice (⅛ of an 8-inch tart dish) about 3 inches wide

18–20 reduced-fat vanilla wafer cookies

1 8-ounce package light cream cheese, softened

¼ cup white sugar

2 mangoes, peeled, seeded, and chopped (about 2 cups)

1 tablespoon lemon juice

1–2 cups blueberries (fresh or frozen)

2 tablespoons powdered sugar for dusting the top of the tart

1. Lay 18–20 vanilla wafer cookies in the bottom of an 8-inch tart dish or pan, flat-side-down.
2. Meanwhile, in a large mixing bowl, beat cream cheese, white sugar, mangoes, and lemon juice on medium speed until mixture is fairly smooth except for small pieces of mango. Spread this over the wafer cookies. Top with blueberries, cover, and refrigerate at least a couple of hours.
3. Dust lightly with powdered sugar before serving

Nutritional Facts (*per serving*): 159 calories, 3 g protein, 24 g carbohydrate, 5.5 g fat (3.4 g saturated fat, 0.1 g monounsaturated fat, 0.2 g polyunsaturated fat, 0.1 g omega-3 fatty acids, 0.1 g omega-6 fatty acids), 13 mg cholesterol, 2 g fiber, 152 mg sodium. Calories from fat: 31 percent.

234 RE vitamin A, 13 mg vitamin C, 0 IU vitamin D, 1.1 IU vitamin E, 0 mcg vitamin B_{12}, 10 mcg folate, 44 mg calcium, 0.5 mcg selenium.

8

If I'm Sweating So Much, Why Aren't I Losing Weight?

Okay ladies, I'm going to give it to you straight! Here are the body weight and shape changes we all have to look forward to after menopause:

- Menopause changes where you put on excess body fat (you will now tend to store it around the waist).
- Fat metabolism appears to change during menopause, making women more likely to store fat and less likely to shed it. This may be caused by lowered levels of estrogen postmenopause.
- We tend to have less lean body mass (muscle), which lowers our metabolic rate—lean muscle mass burns more calories at rest just for maintenance than less lean body mass does.

Not a pretty picture, is it? But I'm an eternal optimist and I have faith that two old sayings will serve us well here: "knowledge is power" and "forewarned is forearmed." In other words, now that we know what to expect (body-size-wise) going into life after peri-menopause, there are various tools and tricks that we can employ in our lives and with our meals to minimize these undesirable body changes.

Namely, we can stave off weight gain (in general and around the middle) by fighting this reduction in metabolic rate and eating defensively. If you haven't yet become a "health nut"—that is, paying attention to what you put in your mouth and whether it nourishes the body or potentially harms the body—now is a pivotal time to start. Although the earlier you start eating healthy, the better, another old saying comes to mind: "better late than never." In this chapter, my aim is to supply you with information and tools about weight loss and weight maintenance so that you will be able to minimize this highly unpopular aspect of menopause.

How to Give Your Metabolism a Boost

Exercise is the best way to keep your weight under control—it may be even more important than what we eat in preventing menopausal weight gain. Some experts recommend regular aerobic exercise, such as brisk walking, 30 minutes a day, while other experts suggest sixty minutes a day. But hold on, you're not getting away that easily. When it comes to muscle and aging, generally the rule is "use it or lose it." And if you want to stop weight gain before it starts, trust me, you'll want to use your muscles. So the ideal exercise plan should include the regular aerobic exercise and some muscle toning and firming exercise as well, such as lifting weights.

Another key way to stimulate our metabolism is to vary our exercise activities and the intensity of these activities by doing several different types of exercise each week. You might take one or two Pilates classes each week, walk several times a week, and do an intense 30-minute muscle-toning workout like Curves several times a week. And if that isn't enough, here's another vital reason to put your exercise program into high gear: Body fat cells are more likely to be burned up at times when additional energy is needed by the body—for example, during exercise.

Pumping Iron

It all comes down to this: The more muscle you have, the more calories (energy) your body will spend in a day, and the more calories you can consume and not gain weight. In a perfect postmenopause world, women would be firming and toning muscle and also participating in regular aerobic exercise. This effort might involve daily 45-minute walks in addition to working out with weights three or four times a week.

Calories Do Count

The harsh reality is that during menopause, even with all this exercise, you may also need to eat less—shaving off perhaps as much as 200–400 calories a day—and exercise more just to maintain your current weight. But for many of us, if we keep an open mind, it is somewhat easy to find a spare 200 calories to cut. How about that daily sugary soda or fancy coffee drink? How about those chips with that sandwich? Those can amount to 200 calories! The key is to cut the foods or drinks that are high in calories but low in important nutrients.

And we can't talk about extra calories without bringing up portion control. If you truly eat when you are hungry and stop when you are comfortable, as you age, your portion sizes may get a little smaller (to compensate for your lower metabolic rate).

Cancel Your Membership in the Clean Plate Club

Some of us are charter members of the Clean Plate Club, started at our dinner tables in the 50s and 60s, when the family rule was that you ate all the food that was put in front of you. It's a habit. Even when we are aware of the "eat when you are hungry; stop when you are comfortable" principle, we still clean our plates. Do not do this anymore. Here's some information on appropriate portion sizes to help you cancel your membership in the Clean Plate Club:

Fact: Larger portions contain more calories.

Fact: Larger portions encourage people to eat more.

In one study, when people were served 2 pounds of lasagna as a first helping, they ended up eating 22 percent more than when they started out with just a half-pound or 1-pound portion. They simply ate what was put before them, so if less was put before them, that's all they ate, and they didn't necessarily want more. Other research found that when portions were larger, women ate 335 more calories per day, and when the portions were doubled, women ate 530 more calories per day.

Walking the Alcohol Minefield

Speaking of cutting extra calories—start at the bar. Let's face it, alcoholic beverages are basically empty calories—calories that don't contribute significant nutritional value. Cutting back on alcohol can really help women after menopause.

Women will often say things like "This dessert is going to go straight to my hips." There should be another common saying: "This beer is going straight to my belly." A gram of alcohol is worth 7 calories (a gram of protein and carbohydrate is worth only 4 calories). And that's not even the worst part. These alcohol calories are mostly "extra" calories, because the body cannot use them as energy in the same way it can use carbohydrates—so they generally get turned into fat. This is not good when you are postmenopausal and trying to keep extra weight off. An 8-ounce serving of red wine, for example, has about 170 calories and 4 grams of carbohydrates, less than 1 gram of protein, and no fat grams to speak of. This means that about 150 of those 170 calories are from alcohol.

So what's a beer-drinking or wine-sipping (and weight-conscious) person to do? Keep in mind that there are several ways to walk through the alcohol minefield without blowing up your healthful, postmenopause intentions:

1. Consider alcoholic beverages a weekly "treat" (instead of a daily ritual), and keep your amounts moderate when you do imbibe (about one drink for women).
2. Don't drink on an empty stomach. This does two things for you. If you enjoy a nice, balanced meal a little bit before you drink or while you drink, you'll be less likely to overconsume alcohol. And second, since you are taking in other nutrients, such as protein and carbs, in the food being absorbed and used as energy, the food will help moderate the negative metabolic effects of the empty calories from alcohol.
3. Make better choices. Simply by choosing certain beers, or light, nonalcoholic, or mixed drinks that use diet sodas or club soda, you can minimize the carb and alcohol calories coming from your cocktail.

Healing the Hurt or Pain in Your Past

Below, you will find the ten keys to taking off weight and keeping it off. However, there is one area that these ten secret weapons don't cover: the emotional and psychological issues that many women have about food. Binge eating is the most common eating disorder and affects about 4 million Americans. Binge eaters frequently and compulsively eat excessive amounts of food, often in secret.

If you would describe yourself as a compulsive eater or someone who frequently overeats, eating to the point of discomfort, I urge you to consider some type of one-on-one therapy (counseling, hypnosis, etc.) as a way to identify and heal the hurt or pain in your past that is causing you to turn to food for comfort.

The key to losing weight does not lie in finding the right fad diet—the key is to eat and exercise for the health of it and let the pounds fall where they may. Learn to eat well for the rest of your life. Here are the secrets to success.

Secret Weapon #1: Got Dairy?

The new National Dairy Council slogan could be, "Got Milk? Lose Weight!" That's right, folks, calcium is in the health spotlight again, but this time it isn't about bones, it's about body fat. New research suggests that lowfat dairy products may be a new weapon to help fight the battle of the bulge. And peri- and postmenopausal women in particular might want to pay attention. The higher a woman's calcium intake, the less chance she has of gaining weight in midlife, according to researcher Dr. Heaney from Creighton University in Omaha.

Increased dairy calcium appears to be a key factor in promoting weight loss (not to mention calcium's ties to preventing osteoporosis, controlling high blood pressure, and potentially reducing the incidence of colon and breast cancer).

Dairy: Weight-Loss Enhancers

High-calcium diets may help slim you down by changing how your body processes fat, according to research from the University of Tennessee. Recent studies suggest that dietary calcium lowers body weight by converting a portion of food energy to heat rather than to stored body fat. When we take dairy products out of our diet we are, in essence, sending our body the signal to make more fat, says Michael Zemel, Ph.D., lead researcher on a study reported in the *American Journal of Clinical Nutrition*. When your body is deprived of calcium, it begins conserving calcium. This mechanism then prompts your body to produce higher levels of a hormone called *calcitriol,* which triggers an increased production of fat cells. Extra calcium in your diet suppresses calcitriol, which leads to the breakdown of more fat, thereby making fat cells leaner and meaner. Zemel estimates that a higher-dairy diet can boost weight loss by as much as 70 percent—and that's no small potatoes!

When you get calcium from lowfat dairy products, you are consuming calcium in its natural environment, in the good company of fellow minerals like magnesium, vitamins, lactose (milk sugars), and protein, some of which may also enhance our fat-burning machinery.

Waist Not Want Not

One of the gifts of menopause is a change in body shape. Word has it the body becomes more likely to store excess fat around the midsection—something I personally find rather unsettling, considering that I am already influenced by a mostly apple-shaped family and have been battling the amazing expanding waist since puberty. Calcium can actually help us with this annoying little side effect of aging as well.

Get this: The dairy participants in the Zemel study lost body fat primarily in the waist. The yogurt-eating study group's waist sizes dropped an average of more than an inch and a half, while their weight dropped an average of 13 pounds, compared to the calcium supplement group, who lost less than half the pounds of the other group and averaged a loss of only a quarter of an inch around the waist. There's a big health bonus for you in these trimmer waists, too: Less weight around the middle means a lower risk of developing heart disease or metabolic syndrome.

Three servings of lowfat dairy products a day would give you the recommended amount of calcium to experience these wonderful weight-loss benefits.

Use It or Lose It

As we age, our bodies naturally start making less lactase (the enzyme that digests lactose, the milk sugar). Your body may also make less lactase if you go through a long period of not consuming dairy products. But don't let being lactose-intolerant stand in your way. If you are lactose-intolerant, you can try:

- consuming smaller quantities of dairy, but having them more often.
- consuming dairy products with food instead of on their own.
- eating dairy products with lower amounts of lactose, such as yogurt and hard cheeses.
- using lactose-free or reduced-lactose products (there are some new, lactose-free milks available).
- using some of the lactaid or lactase enzyme products. The idea here is to add the enzyme to your meal so the lactose sugars are being digested as they usually are in the body.

Secret Weapon #2: A Serving of Soy

Calcium and lowfat dairy products may have some company. Soy may mimic many of the suggested weight-loss benefits of calcium and dairy, according to a new study (*American Journal of Clinical Nutrition,* Dec. 2002). This could be the beginning of a string of research on soy and weight loss, but for now we'll have to wait for more research on soy's weight-loss potential. For lots more info on soy, check out Chapter 2.

Secret Weapon #3: Where's the Water?

Fact: Your body needs water to metabolize stored fat. And most of us want to break down or use excess stored fat, so we should drink lots of water. But what about foods that have lots of water? Some experts say that when people eat foods that have a high water content, they feel fuller longer and tend to consume fewer calories—and this is in addition to the fullness experienced after eating high-fiber foods. Imagine what the water and fiber content of various foods could do together to encourage fullness.

This is great news for fruits and vegetables, which are made up of 80 to 90 percent water. And there are some notoriously high-protein foods that actually contain lots of water, too—eggs and fish are nearly 70 percent water.

Secret Weapon #4: Don't Forget the Fiber

Most Americans need to double their daily amount of fiber. We get about 10–12 grams a day, but we should be getting between 30 and 35 grams. Fiber is the indigestible part of plant food, and since your body doesn't digest, it adds zero calories. Aside from the plethora of health benefits from boosting your daily fiber totals, from a weight-loss/maintenance perspective, fiber expands in your stomach and gives you a sense of fullness, and it will slow down digestion. One study found that people ate smaller lunches after eating higher-fiber breakfasts (the fiber may help lower insulin levels, and insulin helps stimulate your appetite).

Secret Weapon #5: The Big Breakfast Boost

Skipping breakfast is like starting on a long road trip in a car with the fuel gauge almost on empty. By the time you wake up in the morning, your dinner and even dessert from the night before have been digested and the calories (or energy) have been mostly spent. The key is to eat the right blend of foods for breakfast to avoid hunger later. A good, balanced breakfast would include some carbohydrates that contribute fiber and nutrients, and some protein from lowfat dairy, eggs, or lean meats, and some fat from lowfat dairy, eggs, lean meats, or canola oil used to make muffins or to cook hash browns.

When kids skip breakfast, they don't do as well on their schoolwork, especially late in the morning. This makes total sense. Whatever fuel or energy your body had left first thing in the morning is definitely gone by mid- to late morning. Without energy, your muscles don't work as well, and your brain doesn't think as fast.

So the #1 rule to a healthy breakfast is: Don't even think of skipping it. The #2 rule to a healthy breakfast is: Eat a breakfast that isn't too high in sugar and fat, and that isn't too low in nutrition. Many of the breakfast items advertised on television, such as toaster pastries, breakfast bars, and sugary breakfast cereals, are either loaded with fat or sugar. Ask yourself these questions when you are thinking about what to have for breakfast:

- Does my breakfast have something from the milk group or meat group?
  (That would add some protein to your breakfast.)
- Does my breakfast have something from the breads and grains group?
  (The closer to being a bread or grain, the better. Hot oatmeal, for example, has a lot of nutrients and fiber, but Cheerios, a cereal made with a little bit of oats, has a lot less going for it nutritionally.)
- Does my breakfast have something from the fruit group? (High-sugar fruit fillings don't count.) In other words, strawberry Pop-Tarts don't count as fruit, but a waffle topped with fresh or frozen strawberries does.

Secret Weapon #6: Don't Drink Your Calories

Fluids quench your thirst, not hunger—so be careful that you don't spend too many calories quenching your thirst. Some research even suggests that when we drink 100 calories, we will still eat as much later on—as if we hadn't even drunk those calories earlier. And from 1977 to 1998, soft drink consumption increased by more than 60 percent.

Secret Weapon #7: Don't Eat Out As Often

As the number of meals eaten away from home increases, so will your calorie and fat gram tally for the day. Higher amounts of restaurant visits have also been associated with greater body fat levels. Hard to argue with those numbers!

What do you do when you do eat out?

When it comes to eating out and staying on our healthy-eating track, it all comes down to choices, choices, choices. We choose which restaurant or fast-food chain we'll go to. We choose which menu items to order. We choose which condiments and sauces, and how much, are added to our food items. And we choose whether we eat until we are stuffed or just comfortable.

You can still eat healthy when eating out. The following tips will get you started.

- Choose restaurants or fast-food outlets that are known for healthful eating options.
- Be sure to choose some of the lighter menu options.
- Try to work some fresh fruit and vegetables into your meal. Although only oven-baked, lowfat french fries count as a serving of vegetables.
- Eat reasonable serving sizes (not those supersized portions many restaurants serve—you can always take half your meal home in a doggie bag!)
- Use lower-calorie condiments, such as mustard, ketchup, and reduced-fat salad dressing, instead of mayonnaise, tartar sauce, and high-calorie salad dressing. A lower-fat version of mayonnaise (mayonnaise blended with a lot of fat-free sour cream) is used as a mayo substitute in several recipes in this book.

Secret Weapon #8: Get Fruity

The amount of fruit you eat in a day may contribute to weight loss, suggests a new Brazilian study. The women who ate three apples or three pears a day lost more weight than the group instructed to eat oats three times a day. And as luck would have it, obesity levels are the lowest among those who eat seven or more servings of fruits and vegetables a day. When one study compared the intake of consumers with the healthiest diets to consumers with the least healthy diets, researchers found that the biggest single difference was the amount of fruit they ate (the healthiest diets being the ones with the highest fruit intake).

Secret Weapon #9: Soup It Up!

Start a meal with soup, but not the high-fat variety. Studies suggest that when you do this, you tend to eat less at that meal and later in the day.

Along the same water principle, it follows that soup really is "good food." Soup is known for giving us a fuller feeling longer, so we might tend to eat fewer calories overall in a meal if we start the meal with a cup of clear-broth- or tomato-based soup, not higher-calorie/fat cream-based soup.

Secret Weapon #10: Choose Your Carbs Wisely

Make sure most of your carbohydrates contribute fiber and important nutrients (phytochemicals, vitamins, and minerals, etc.)—the less refined and processed, the better. If you think about some of the most nutritious foods on the planet—fruits, vegetables, beans, and whole grains—they are all rich in carbohydrates! Just because Americans have been making poor carbohydrate choices as part of their effort to eat a lower-fat diet doesn't mean you throw the baby out with the bathwater and blame *all* carbohydrates. Go out of your way to chose whole grains, beans, fruits, and vegetables whenever possible.

12 Habits of Successful Weight Maintenance

Anyone can lose weight, experts say, but very few will be able to keep it off over the years. Those of us who have ridden the fad-diet roller coaster more than a few times can attest to that. So the billion-dollar question becomes: What makes the difference between those who do successfully keep it off and those who aren't as lucky? Is it really luck, or is there something we can all do?

If the National Weight Control Registry can't answer that question, no one can. The Registry has been tracking 3,000 people who have successfully lost an average of 66 pounds and kept it off for 5.5 years. Obviously, if family members are nurturing and supportive, a person stands a better chance of losing weight permanently. But the Registry has also definitely seen some patterns in healthy food habits in the people who have maintained their weight loss over years and years. When the Registry studied what was going on with the people who were regaining their lost weight, they found two distinct themes: decreases in physical activity and increases in fat intake.

Of course, it also depends on whom you ask. If you look at a study in the *International Journal of Obesity,* the successful maintainers had these characteristics in common: They dieted for longer periods, were originally motivated to lose weight for psychological reasons (improving self-esteem or overcoming depression), and reported eating healthy food more often than the less successful dieters.

The other words of advice from a recent weight-loss study is, hang in there, because it eventually does get easier. This study found that the longer a person maintains their weight loss, the easier that maintenance becomes (Mary L. Klem, Ph.D., University of Pittsburgh School of Medicine). How much time are we talking about? Once people have lost weight and kept it off for two years, they tend to be fairly stable thereafter, assures Arthur Frank, M.D., Medical Director of the George Washington University Weight Management Program.

No one says it is going to be easy. To lose weight permanently, you must make a commitment to gradually adopt a healthier way of life for the rest of your life. It sounds rather ominous, I know, but if this new way of living entails eating great-tasting food (including many healthier versions of your favorite foods) and an hour a day of exercise that you actually enjoy with people you look forward to seeing, it can actually be, dare I say it, pleasurable. The following are the twelve habits that people who successfully maintain their weight loss have in common.

Habit #1: They Eat a Low-Fat, High-Carb Diet

Less than 1 percent of the National Weight Control Registry's successful "losers" ate low-carb diets for weight maintenance, including higher-fiber carbohydrates, such as whole grains, beans, fruits, and vegetables. Most ate the low-fat, high-carb way to maintain their weight loss, even if they lost the weight with a different type of diet. Generally people in the

Registry say they get about 56 percent of their calories from carbohydrates, 19 percent from protein, and 25 percent from fat. When about 25 percent of your calories come from fat (preferably using the better fats, i.e., monounsaturated fats like olive oil and canola oil and omega-3s from fish and canola oil, and some helpful polyunsaturated fats found in nuts and other plant foods), you are taking in enough fat to encourage a feeling of satisfaction but not too much fat (since fat is a major contributor to calories).

New research adds more reasons to eat a lower-fat diet. Eating a lowfat diet allows you to avoid the increase in levels of *ghrelin* (a newly discovered hormone secreted by the stomach that stimulates appetite) that you normally see when someone is restricting their calories, according to a new study. The researchers also noted that dietary fat restriction often decreases excessive fat in the body without increasing appetite.

Habit #2: They Eat Breakfast Every Day

People on the Registry's success list usually never skip breakfast. Skipping meals in general isn't a good idea, because skipping meals usually means you'll be starving later, and when many people get that hungry, they are more likely to either overeat when they do finally eat and/or eat unhealthful foods.

Habit #3: They Eat Five Small Meals Throughout the Day

Eating more often, but smaller amounts at a time, is a good idea for every single American but can be particularly helpful for women in the midst of menopause. Small meals eaten every few hours translates into more stable blood sugar levels and more energy throughout your day. Eating smaller, more frequent meals is helpful for appetite control, too. It makes sense that people who eat smaller, more frequent meals are less likely to overeat at any meal. Larger meals also flood your bloodstream with larger amounts of fat, protein, and carb calories, and those excess calories have to go somewhere—so many are converted to body fat for energy storage.

Habit #4: They Weigh Themselves About Once a Week

Seventy-five percent of the people being tracked by the National Weight Control Registry weigh themselves once a week. Perhaps this weekly weigh-in serves as an early-warning system that they are getting off track. I prefer to use what I call "the tight-jean test." I use a pair of jeans as my weight-gain gauge. I like this better, because it stops you from being "pound" obsessed and moves you more toward how your clothes fit and feel.

Habit #5: They Don't Deprive Themselves of Favorite Foods; They Enjoy Them in Moderation

Don't fall for food bans. Being too strict can make it hard to stick to a healthy eating plan. And forcing yourself to give up certain foods completely can lead to bingeing—and bingeing can lead to overeating, guilty feelings, and an array of potentially disordered eating practices.

Habit #6: They Shy Away from Sugar and Bring On the Fiber-Rich Carbs

Refined and processed carbohydrate-rich foods are digested quickly and can produce ups and downs in your blood sugar levels. Substituting whole grains and high-fiber foods can increase stomach satisfaction, and eating plenty of water- and fiber-filled fruits and vegetables can help make you feel full on fewer calories.

Habit #7: No Bells and Whistles Required

Consumer Reports surveyed 32,000 dieters and found that the majority of people who had kept the extra pounds off for more than a year (83 percent) did it without any gimmicks. Just 14 percent of the people who kept the weight off for more than five years ever signed up with the big dieting program giants or other commercial diet programs. Even fewer used meal replacement shakes or pills.

Habit #8: Exercise, Exercise, Exercise

Many National Weight Control Registry participants exercise for about an hour a day—burning about 2,700 calories a week. But don't let that hour-a-day scare you. Many of the Registry participants exercise a little at a time throughout the day, and many use walking as their major method of exercising. Successful dieters who tried exercising three or more times a week ranked it as their #1 dieting strategy (eight out of ten of the successful dieters), according to the *Consumer Reports* survey. Walking was the most popular form of exercise for long-term weight-loss success, but close to 30 percent also added weight lifting to their routine to increase calorie-burning muscle mass.

Habit #9: They Changed Their Lifestyle

Lifestyle changes have proven to work for weight loss, asserts Catherine D. DeAngelis, M.D., MPH, the editor of the *Journal of the American Medical Association*. If your past lifestyle of overeating unhealthy foods and under-exercising got you into this overweight mess to begin with, wouldn't it make sense to change your lifestyle not just to lose the weight but to keep it off for good? Sounds simple, but those of you who have tried to change old habits know it is anything but. Keep in mind that the more you practice a certain behavior, the easier it becomes, until eventually you do it without even thinking about it.

Habit #10: The Internet Was Their Weight-Loss Friend

Many women say they get valuable around-the-clock support from website weight-loss community boards—this type of help, 24-7, is not easily duplicated with books, weekly group meetings, or occasional consultations with a dietitian. Dr. Deborah Tate, Ph.D., a researcher with Brown University, found that people who augmented a weight-loss program with Internet tools such as food journals and message boards lost three times as much weight in a six-month period as those who didn't. Tate also found that dieters who used an Internet weight-loss program but also had regular e-mail consultations with a dietitian lost twice as much weight as those who simply logged on to a diet website and tracked their daily food and exercise.

Habit #11: They Recovered Quickly from Lapses

People who have maintained their weight loss sometimes have lapses, but the trick is not to dwell on it and dig yourself deeper in a hole but to get right back on the horse, eating sensibly and exercising as soon as possible, says Arthur Frank, M.D., Medical Director of the George Washington University Weight Management Program in Washington.

Habit #12: They Kept a Food Journal

Recording what you eat and drink in a food journal will help you learn about your eating habits so you can make healthful changes and will allow you to identify patterns (for example, a correlation between certain emotions and increased food intake).

Recipes to Keep You Fit at Fifty

Don't get me wrong, all the recipes in this book can help keep you fit at fifty. Most are lower in fat and most include carbohydrates that contain fiber and nutrients. Many of the recipes feature lowfat dairy ingredients and/or soy, and you'll find a few soup recipes in other chapters as well. So for the recipes in this chapter, I focused on recipes for quick, high-fiber breakfasts and threw an extra soup recipe in for the heck of it.

Ham & Cheese Breakfast Pocket

These are fun little breakfast sandwiches to make quickly in a nonstick frying pan or skillet. What makes them fun? They look like a pocket, and you can hold them easily in your hand, too. If you want to jazz them up a bit, a teaspoon or two of the Scallion-Soy Cream Cheese (recipe on page 145) tastes great spread on top of the ham.

Makes 2 pockets • Serving size: 2 pockets

2 slices whole-wheat or whole-grain sliced bread (about 38 grams per slice and 3 grams of fiber per slice)

1 ounce reduced-fat cheddar, jack, Swiss, Jarlsberg, or other reduced-fat cheese, grated or sliced

1 ounce extra-lean sliced ham (brown-sugar, honey, or smoked)

1. Heat a medium nonstick frying pan or skillet over medium heat. Lightly spray one side of the bread slices with canola oil cooking spray. Lay the bread slices, oil-side down, in the pan.
2. Evenly distribute the cheese and ham on the top of the bread slices. When the bottom of the bread is nicely brown, flip with spatula and brown the other side. Enjoy!

Nutritional Facts (*per serving*): 254 calories, 19 g protein, 27 g carbohydrate, 8.5 g fat (4 g saturated fat, 3 g monounsaturated fat, 0.8 g polyunsaturated fat, 0.1 g omega-3 fatty acids, 0.7 g omega-6 fatty acids), 28 mg cholesterol, 4 g fiber, 849 mg sodium. Calories from fat: 30 percent.

54 RE vitamin A, 0 mg vitamin C, 5 IU vitamin D, 1 IU vitamin E, 0.5 mcg vitamin B$_{12}$, 32 mcg folate, 250 mg calcium, 25 mcg selenium.

Scallion-Soy Cream Cheese

I'm a bagel lover from way back, and I'm always looking for fun ways to eat them. This is a yummy bagel spread that will wake you up with flavorful scallions and will get a dose of soy into your morning to boot. Plus, you'll get 2 milligrams of isoflavones per serving!

Makes 1⅛ cup • Serving size: ⅛ cup

1 cup soy cream cheese (i.e., 1 8-ounce container of Veggie Cream Cheese by Galaxy Nutritional Foods)

⅓ cup chopped scallions (white and part of green)

Salt and pepper to taste (optional)

1. Add soy cream cheese and chopped scallions to a mini food processor or small mixing bowl and beat until well blended. Add salt and pepper to taste if desired.
2. Spoon into a small serving bowl, cover tightly with plastic wrap, and store in the refrigerator until needed. (The spread will keep nicely for several days.)

Note: If you can't find soy cream cheese in your supermarket, you can blend ½ cup of light (block) cream cheese with ½ cup of soft or silken tofu instead. It will be a little less firm compared to the soy cream cheese, but it will still taste delicious and will spread nicely on bagels. (Just eat them as open-faced bagels with the spread on top of each half.)

Nutritional Facts *(per ⅛ cup serving)*: 46 calories, 2 g protein, 2 g carbohydrate, 2.7 g fat (n/a g saturated fat, n/a g monounsaturated fat, n/a g polyunsaturated fat, n/a g omega-3 fatty acids, n/a g omega-6 fatty acids), 0 mg cholesterol, 0.1 g fiber, 196 mg sodium. Calories from fat: 52 percent.

Honey—Wheat Bran Muffins

This muffin contains everything you would expect it to have: wheat bran and raisins. But it has a little something extra—canola oil, which is high in monounsaturated fat and plant-derived omega-3s, and it has some soy flour. If you don't want to use soy flour, you can add ¼ cup of ground flaxseeds instead, or increase the white flour to 1 cup. You might enjoy these muffins with a little spoon of Cinna-Soy Butter (recipe on page 147).

Makes 12 muffin cups • Serving size: one muffin

1½ cups wheat bran

1⅛ cups lowfat buttermilk

3 tablespoons canola oil

3 tablespoons honey

1 large egg (a high-omega-3 egg, if available)

⅓ cup brown sugar, packed

1 teaspoon vanilla extract

¾ cup unbleached white flour

¼ cup soy flour

1 teaspoon baking soda

1 teaspoon baking powder

½ teaspoon salt

½ cup raisins

1. Preheat the oven to 375 degrees. Line a muffin pan with paper or foil muffin liners.
2. Place wheat bran and buttermilk in a mixing bowl and let stand for 10 minutes.
3. Add oil, honey, egg, brown sugar, and vanilla to bran mixture and beat on low to blend well. Scrape the sides of the bowl halfway through mixing.
4. Place flours, baking soda, baking powder, and salt in a medium-size bowl and blend well with whisk or fork. Add the flour mixture to the wheat-bran mixture all at once and beat on low to blend together, scraping sides of bowl halfway through mixing.
5. Fold in raisins and spoon (about ¼ cup of batter) into each muffin cup. Bake 15–20 minutes, or until toothpick inserted into the center of a muffin comes out clean.

Nutritional Facts *(per muffin)*: 158 calories, 5 g protein, 27 g carbohydrate, 4.9 g fat (0.6 g saturated fat, 2.3 g monounsaturated fat, 1.1 g polyunsaturated fat, 0.3 g omega-3 fatty acids, 0.8 g omega-6 fatty acids), 19 mg cholesterol, 4 g fiber, 277 mg sodium. Calories from fat: 28 percent.

7 RE vitamin A, 0.4 mg vitamin C, 2.2 IU vitamin D, 1.3 IU vitamin E, 0 mcg vitamin B_{12}, 16 mcg folate, 62 mg calcium, 4.1 mcg selenium.

Cinna-Soy Butter

Every little bit helps, and this is yet another way to work a little soy into your breakfast. Use this lightly spiced soy butter on almost anything: toast, pancakes, waffles, breakfast rolls, or muffins. If you don't want to make quite this much, just cut the recipe in half and use an electric mixer instead of a mini food processor.

Makes 1 cup (16 tablespoons) • Serving size: one tablespoon

½ cup no- or low-trans-fat margarine (for example Land O' Lakes Fresh Buttery Taste Spread, or Smart Balance) or butter, softened

½ cup soft or silken tofu (light or regular)
3 tablespoons powdered sugar
¾ teaspoon ground cinnamon
Dash ground nutmeg (optional)

1. Add margarine or butter, tofu, sugar, cinnamon, and nutmeg to a mini food processor and pulse until light and creamy. If you don't have a mini food processor, you can use an electric mixer and beat in small bowl on high for 1–2 minutes.
2. Add to a custard cup, cover tightly with plastic wrap, and store in the refrigerator until needed. (The Cinna-Soy Butter will keep for several days.)

Nutritional Facts (*per tablespoon with regular tofu*): 62 calories, 1 g protein, 2 g carbohydrate, 5.8 g fat (0.8 g saturated fat, 2.8 g monounsaturated fat, 1.7 g polyunsaturated fat, 0.3 g omega-3 fatty acids, 1 g omega-6 fatty acids), 0 mg cholesterol, 0 g fiber, 48 mg sodium. Calories from fat: 84 percent.

50 RE vitamin A, 0 mg vitamin C, 0 IU vitamin D, 0 IU vitamin E, 0 mcg vitamin B_{12}, 5 mcg folate, 12 mg calcium, 1 mcg selenium.

Sun-dried Tomato–Pesto Soy Spread

Makes 1 cup • Serving size: ⅛ cup

1 cup fresh basil leaves, rinsed, drained, and packed

⅛ cup chopped softened sun-dried tomatoes (if using the bottled sun-dried tomatoes, drain well before adding)

1½ teaspoons garlic, minced or crushed

⅛ teaspoon salt (optional)

2 tablespoons pine nuts or walnuts, toasted

1 tablespoon olive oil

1 8-ounce container (about 1 cup) soy cream cheese (for example, veggie Cream Cheese by Galaxy Nutritional Foods)

1. Place basil, tomatoes, garlic, salt (if desired), nuts, olive oil, and soy cream cheese in a mini food processor. (If using a regular-size food processor or blender, you will need to double the recipe.) Pulse until a nice puree forms.

2. Spoon into a custard cup, cover tightly with plastic wrap, and store in the refrigerator until needed. (The spread will keep well for a few days.)

Note: If you can't find soy cream cheese in your supermarket, you can blend ½ cup of light (block) cream cheese with ½ cup of soft or silken tofu instead. It will be a little less firm compared to the soy cream cheese, but it will still taste delicious and will spread nicely on bagels. (Just eat them as open-faced bagels with the spread on top of each half.)

Nutritional Facts *(per serving)*: 81 calories, 3 g protein, 3 g carbohydrate, 5.5 g fat (0.4 g saturated fat, 1.8 g monounsaturated fat, 0.6 g polyunsaturated fat, 0.1 g omega-3 fatty acids, 0.5 g omega-6 fatty acids), 0 mg cholesterol, 0.5 g fiber, 264 mg sodium. Calories from fat: 61 percent.

21 RE vitamin A, 2 mg vitamin C, 0 IU vitamin D, 0.5 IU vitamin E, 0 mcg vitamin B_{12}, 5 mcg folate, 110 mg calcium, 0.5 mcg selenium.

Plus: 2 mg isoflavones per serving!

Make-Ahead French Toast

How can you resist a breakfast recipe that you make a day ahead of time, then just pop in the oven in the morning? The French toast looks and tastes great topped with fresh fruit.

Makes 6 servings • Serving size: 1 6-inch slice

3 eggs, lightly beaten (preferably high-
    omega-3 eggs)
½ cup egg substitute (i.e., Egg Beaters)
1½ cups lowfat milk
1 cup fat-free half-and-half
1½ teaspoons vanilla extract
6 1-inch-thick slices of whole-wheat bread or
    12 ½-inch-thick slices (about 1 pound)

2 tablespoons butter or no- or low-trans-
    fat margarine, melted
1 teaspoon ground cinnamon
½ cup maple syrup or reduced-calorie
    pancake syrup
½ cup chopped pecans

1. In a large bowl, whisk together eggs, egg substitute, milk, half-and-half, and vanilla. Pour 1 cup of the egg mixture into a lightly greased 9x13-inch baking dish. Dip bread slices into remaining egg mixture and place in the prepared dish. (If you bought pre-sliced bread, you can lay 2 ½-inch-thick slices on top of each other to make 1-inch stacks. Drizzle 1 cup of the remaining egg mixture over the top of the bread slices and cover the dish well. Refrigerate overnight.

2. The next morning: Preheat oven to 350 degrees.

3. In a small bowl, combine butter, cinnamon, maple syrup, and pecans. Spoon mixture over the bread.

4. Bake until golden, about 40 minutes. Let stand 5 minutes before serving.

Nutritional Facts *(per serving)*: 415 calories, 17 g protein, 53 g carbohydrate, 16 g fat (4.5 g saturated fat, 7.3 g monounsaturated fat, 3.2 g polyunsaturated fat, 0.2 g omega-3 fatty acids, 3 g omega-6 fatty acids), 120 mg cholesterol, 5 g fiber, 489 mg sodium. Calories from fat: 34 percent.

190 RE vitamin A, 1 mg vitamin C, 85 IU vitamin D, 2.3 IU vitamin E, 0.8 mcg vitamin B_{12}, 60 mcg folate, 284 mg calcium, 31 mcg selenium.

Lighter French Onion Soup

In this recipe we reduced the sodium and brought the fat content down a notch or two, while also switching to a high-monounsaturated fat, which all sounds like it isn't going to taste so great—but it really does. This soup is so satisfying that it can actually be the meal instead of just starting it off.
Makes 6 servings • Serving size: about 1 cup

3 ounces (¾ cup) reduced-fat Jarlsberg or Swiss cheese, grated (½ cup of grated Gruyère can be substituted)

4 tablespoons Parmesan cheese, shredded

1 tablespoon olive oil

4 large yellow onions, thinly sliced lengthwise

1 tablespoon minced garlic

2 bay leaves

12 ounces (1½ cups) nonalcoholic or light beer (substitute apple cider, if desired)

½ teaspoon salt (optional)

½ teaspoon freshly ground pepper

¼ cup Madeira (or similar) wine (substitute broth if desired)

2 cups low-sodium chicken or beef broth

1 10½-ounce can condensed beef consommé

Soup croutons (recipe follows)

1. Combine the Jarlsberg and Parmesan cheeses; set aside. Heat the olive oil in a large nonstick soup pot or saucepan over medium-low heat. Add the onions, garlic, and bay leaves, and cook until the onions begin to brown.

2. Add ½ cup of the beer and cook until the onions begin to caramelize. Add the salt (if desired) and pepper, and continue stirring another minute. Add the wine and the remaining 1 cup beer, and cook until the liquid is reduced by half. Add the broth and consommé, cover, and simmer for 30 minutes. Adjust the seasoning if necessary and remove the bay leaves.

3. Preheat the broiler. Ladle the soup into ovenproof bowls, float 1 crouton (recipe follows) on top of each, and sprinkle with the cheese mixture. Set the bowls on a baking sheet and place under the broiler until the cheese is lightly browned and bubbling (the cheese can also be melted in the microwave).

Soup Croutons

6 slices sourdough or French bread,
    sliced on the diagonal

2 tablespoons Parmesan cheese,
    shredded or grated

1. Preheat oven to 325 degrees. Coat both sides of the bread with olive oil cooking spray. Place on a cookie sheet and sprinkle the tops of the slices with Parmesan cheese. Bake until crisp and golden brown, about 15 minutes (check often, so the croutons don't burn).

Nutritional Facts *(per serving, including soup croutons)*: 350 calories, 16 g protein, 48 g carbohydrate, 8.8 g fat (3.5 g saturated fat, 3.7 g monounsaturated fat, 0.8 g polyunsaturated fat, 0.1 g omega-3 fatty acids, 0.7 g omega-6 fatty acids), 13 mg cholesterol, 4 g fiber, 1,000 mg sodium. Calories from fat: 23 percent.

36 RE vitamin A, 8 mg vitamin C, 2 IU vitamin D, 1.1 IU vitamin E, 0.2 mcg vitamin B_{12}, 84 mcg folate, 257 mg calcium, 23 mcg selenium.

9.

Boost Your Bones Naturally

When the topic of being overweight comes up, the news regarding health is usually negative. But when it comes to your bones, finally there is a health benefit to the so-called fat gene. That's right, if you are built on the sturdy side, you are less at risk of developing osteoporosis, because the more weight you carry around, the more weight is bearing on your bones, even while doing the simplest of exercises, such as walking, gardening, or housework. And the more weight bearing on your bones, the more your bones are stimulated. My family tree is filled with mostly apple-shaped people—and you would be hard-pressed to find someone in my family with osteoporosis.

In this chapter, though, thin or not, we are going to find out what we can do to boost the bones we have without hormone replacement therapy, because all women need to pay attention to this risk. Getting proper nutrition along with enough calcium and exercise is crucial to protecting our bones after menopause, especially for those of us opting not to go on HRT.

OSTEOPOROSIS RISK FACTORS YOU CAN CHANGE	RISK FACTORS YOU CAN'T DO ANYTHING ABOUT
Cigarette smoking: Smoking results in a faster rate of bone loss by interfering with calcium absorption and lowering estrogen levels.	Having a first-degree relative (a parent or sibling) with an age-related fracture, such as a hip fracture.
A diet low in calcium and vitamin D: Including 1200–1500 milligrams of calcium and 400–800 IU of vitamin D in your daily diet is a good idea for women as they age. In teens and younger women, these positive dietary changes will increase bone strength, which will provide a better baseline when natural bone loss begins.	Being Caucasian or Asian
Using anticonvulsants and glucocorticoid medications. These are medications for seizures and chronic inflammatory diseases, such as certain types of arthritis or intestinal diseases. Ask your doctor whether you can take an alternative medication that won't compromise your bone density. If you need these medications, it is crucial to take them, But try to reduce your osteoporosis risk by even more vigilance with diet and exercise.	Being elderly: The older you are, the greater your risk of developing osteoporosis. Osteoporosis is responsible for more than 1.5 million fractures annually in America.
Excessive alcohol intake: Defined as more than seven drinks per week, excessive alcohol use has been associated with an increased risk of falls and a decrease in bone mineral density.	
Exercising: Weight-bearing exercise (such as low-impact aerobics, jogging, strength training, tennis, dancing, and walking) can help build stronger bones and muscles and can be used to increase strength, flexibility, and balance. But high-impact exercise like running and high-impact aerobics appear to provide the most bone-building stimulation. The more stress to the bones, the stronger the bones become. However, you may need to find a balance between vigorous and moderate exercise to protect your joints and prevent injury.	Having certain medical disorders: hormonal disorders (such as hyperthyroidism), neoplastic disorders (such as cancer), and connective tissue disorders (such as lupus).
Body weight less than 127 pounds: For once, being a little heavier actually helps!	If you have had an organ transplant in your life.

Source: *Journal of Midwifery & Women's Health,* Jan. 2003, Volume 48, Number 1. "Pharmacotherapeutics for Osteoporosis Prevention and Treatment," Michele Davidson, CNM, Ph.D.

What Is Osteoporosis?

Osteoporosis is defined as a progressive systemic disease characterized by low bone density and deterioration of bone tissue with a consequent increase in bone fragility and susceptibility to fracture, which basically means that if you develop osteoporosis, your bones are weakening and getting brittle. As bones lose calcium and other minerals, they become more porous; these little holes make bones more susceptible to breaks. Bone loss begins sometime between 30 and 35 years of age and rapidly accelerates immediately after menopause.

Are You At Risk?

There are a handful of risk factors for osteoporosis that we can do nothing about, and a handful of risk factors that we have the power to change. Check out the list on p. 154, note the risk factors that relate to you, and make a commitment to change them. Do it for your bones!

Note: Some people may need to control their risk of osteoporosis with medication such as calcitonin, bisphosphonates, and selective estrogen receptor modulators. Be sure to discuss your options with your doctor.

OSTEOPOROSIS FAST FACTS
- An estimated 8 million American women have osteoporosis, with another 18 million at risk due to low bone mass.
- Osteoporosis is referred to as a "silent" disease, because you can't feel your bones becoming weaker.
- Symptoms generally do not occur until after the disease has progressed to the point where risk of fracture is very high.
- In the United States, osteoporosis causes more than 1.5 million fractures each year. The fractures are usually in the spine, hip, or wrist.
- Osteoporosis is most common in postmenopausal Caucasian women (although it is also common in Asian women). An estimated 21 to 30 percent of postmenopausal Caucasian women have osteoporosis, and an additional 54 percent have low bone mass.
- Osteoporosis is irreversible but may be prevented by maximizing peak bone mass in your teens and 20s in order to keep your bones strong during the natural periods of

bone loss—namely, menopause and aging. Proper diet in later life can help prevent the rapid bone loss that takes place soon after menopause.

What Does All This Have to Do with Estrogen and HRT?

The estrogen in our body enhances bone formation, which explains why postmenopausal women, whose bodies are no longer producing large amounts of estrogen, represent the most common risk group for osteoporosis. As estrogen levels decrease, bone loss accelerates.

Although hormone replacement therapy helps prevent osteoporosis by decreasing the rate of bone loss, there is no evidence that it is an effective treatment for existing osteoporosis. The Women's Health Initiative Study demonstrated that women taking hormone replacement therapy did reduce hip and clinical vertebral fracture rates by one-third compared to women taking a placebo. But interestingly, the researchers of the study recommended alternative prevention and treatment strategies for osteoporosis in order to avoid the increase in breast cancer that goes along with the hormone replacement therapy. Some of those strategies are what the rest of this chapter will cover, so keep reading!

How to Prevent Rapid Bone Loss During and After Menopause

So what can a 50-something woman knee-deep in hot flashes do to preserve the bone she has left? Let's start with the obvious diet factor: calcium. It all comes down to calcium *in* and calcium *out*. You want to make sure you get enough calcium coming *in* (via the foods you choose), and you want to make sure a minimal amount goes *out* unabsorbed (through urine). You want your body to absorb as much as possible through the intestines.

In order to do this, it's important to know which foods or food components are calcium absorption enhancers that help our bodies absorb the maximum calcium through digestion in the intestines, and which foods or food components are calcium depleters that encourage calcium loss via the kidneys and urine or that discourage calcium absorption from food sources in the intestinal tract.

What Are the Calcium Absorption Enhancers, and Where Can I Get Some?

Vitamin D

Vitamin D builds strong bones in two ways: It improves the amount of calcium that gets absorbed in the intestines and it is also required for normal bone metabolism.

The Dietary Reference Intake (DRI, 1998) for Vitamin D is 400 IU/day (or 10 mcg/day) for women fifty-one to seventy years old, and 600 IU/day (or 15 mcg/day) for women age seventy-one and older. Your body makes vitamin D in your skin with the help of ultraviolet light, but as you age, your body makes less and less of it. The following are a few foods that contain vitamin D naturally.

- fish liver oils (1,360 IU per tablespoon)
- oysters, cooked (640 IU per 3.5 ounces)
- mackerel, canned (360 IU per 3.5 ounces)
- most fish (88 IU per 3.5 ounces)
- egg (26 IU per egg)

You can also find vitamin D in vitamin D–fortified milks, some yogurts, some margarines, and some breakfast cereals. Check the labels to be sure. For example, the label on the lowfat milk in my refrigerator (an organic store brand) states that it contains 25 percent of the daily amount of vitamin D, approximately 100 IU.

Phytoestrogens

Phytoestrogens (plant compounds structurally similar to estrogen) are food components that are gaining more and more attention in bone research, which might help explain why vegans fare so much better bone-wise than one might expect. Plant estrogens possibly suppress the removal of calcium from the bones. Results of animal studies are promising; we'll know more in the years to come. Scientists are just beginning to learn of phytoestrogens' potent positive effect in protecting bone mineral density in postmenopausal women.

The three phytoestrogens being studied are isoflavones, lignans, and coumestans. Soy contains both isoflavones and lignans, and flaxseed is one of the richest sources of lignans.

You'll find these phytoestrogens in lots of fruits and vegetables, too, including apples asparagus, beets, bell peppers, broccoli stems, cabbage, carrots, cauliflower, cucumbers, grapefruit, grapes, lettuce, onions, oranges, pears, raspberries, strawberries, sweet potatoes, and turnips. Whole-wheat products contain lignans, too. You'll find recipes containing these high-powered plant foods throughout this book.

Magnesium

A lack of the mineral magnesium may be an important risk factor for developing osteoporosis, particularly in postmenopausal women. Magnesium helps your bones by increasing calcium absorption in the intestines; it helps the body use vitamin D, which also helps your bones. It also has a role in making and maintaining strong bones. In fact, about half of the body's magnesium does exactly that.

The Dietary Reference Intake for magnesium is 320 mg/day for women age 31 and older. You can find magnesium in many plant foods, such as nuts, seeds, and beans (including soybeans and soy products such as tofu), dark green vegetables like broccoli and spinach, and potatoes. Whole-grain foods, meats, seafood, and milk contain smaller amounts.

What Are the Calcium Depleters?

Sodium, caffeine, high amounts of protein, and alcohol are substances that you eat or drink that, especially in large amounts, can deplete your body of calcium by increasing the amount of calcium in the urine and decreasing the amount of calcium absorbed in the intestines after meals. Obviously, the moral to this story is not to overdo sodium, caffeine, and alcohol, and to avoid high-protein diets in favor of a diet emphasizing fruits and vegetables, whole grains, and beans, balanced with (if you are not a vegetarian) fish, lean meats, and lowfat dairy products.

High-Protein = Low Bone Density?

High-protein diets are no friend to your bones—yet one more reason why you shouldn't eat a high-protein diet. According to Dr. Linda Massey, a researcher and calcium and protein expert with Washington State University, following very high-protein diets for a long time, longer than three months, is likely to be associated with increased bone loss. Dr. Massey defines "high-protein" as 1.5 grams protein per kilogram of body weight or 50 percent more than the Recommended Daily Amount for protein. And a "very high" protein diet is 2 grams protein per kilogram of body weight or two times the Recommended Daily Amount for protein. People who eat high amounts of animal protein over time tend to have a lower amount of bone formation, which is likely to lead to a decrease in bone density. How does the protein you eat affect the bones in your body?

When the body breaks down dietary protein, metabolic by-products, including several types of acids, are created. The body neutralizes these acids with citrate and carbonate from the bones. The amount of calcium lost in the urine increases as the amount of dietary protein increases. Plants such as grains and legumes have something going for them, though: They contain high amounts of potassium, and potassium helps decrease urinary calcium. Milk products can help lessen this effect, too. The high amount of calcium in milk and milk products helps compensate for the calcium that will be lost in the urine due to the digestion/absorption of the protein in milk.

Got Calcium?

We've been talking a lot about the nutrients that enhance or deplete calcium. Now it's time to get down to that king of the bones, calcium. Getting enough calcium in your diet is so important. Here's why:

In general, calcium supplements or high food intake of calcium in postmenopausal women improves bone mineral density and reduces bone loss and fractures.

Getting extra calcium in your diet will also help prevent the bone loss that normally accompanies weight reduction.

During the late postmenopausal period, calcium is more effective at slowing bone loss. I guess it's a "better late than never" scenario.

In 2001, the National Academy of Science revised the recommended amount of calcium required to reflect the wealth of scientific research on the role of calcium in the diet. The latest recommendations are:

Males, age 19–50:	1,000 mg/day
Females, age 51–70+	1,200 mg/day
Pregnant and Lactating females:	1,000 mg/day

The National Institutes of Health recommends that postmenopausal women between the ages of fifty and sixty-four who are not on estrogen or hormone replacement therapy, and all women over sixty-five, consume 1,500 milligrams of calcium a day (1,000 milligrams a day is recommended for postmenopausal women who are taking estrogen). This is a tall order, because barely half of all American women are even reaching the previous goal of 800 milligrams a day. Note: If you have had calcium-containing kidney stones, you should check first with your health-care practitioner on this and other calcium advice.)

Supplements

Clearly, getting as much of the nutrients you need from the foods you eat is best. But some of us may not be reaching those recommended daily amounts, so some type of supplement may be in order. If you are thinking about supplementing your diet with calcium or vitamin D, here are some helpful hints:

1. Rhubarb, tea, and chocolate contain calcium-binding oxalate, but they do not contribute any calcium. They can block the absorption of calcium, so to play it safe, wait two hours after eating a food containing oxalate before taking your supplement.
2. Calcium absorption is best when your calcium supplement is taken with some food. Consider taking your supplement with a light mid-morning or afternoon snack.

3. Your body can't absorb more than 500–600 milligrams of calcium at a time, so a single daily dose of 1,200 milligrams, for example, would not be helpful. Divide the dose over the course of the day if your doctor has recommended that you take more than 600 milligrams a day.

4. USP is the seal of the United States Pharmacopeia, which is there to ensure buyers of uniformity and quality in manufacturing standards among vitamin capsules or tablets. Only use supplements with the USP seal on the package.

5. Read the label so you know exactly what you are buying.

6. Avoid calcium supplements that contain dolomite or bone meal—they may contain very small amounts of lead and other metals that can be harmful.

7. Your calcium supplement should not be your only important source of calcium. Try to work some high-calcium foods into your daily diet, too.

8. Drink plenty of liquids with your calcium supplement to avoid constipation (water works best).

Walking Your Way to Better Bones

Weight-bearing exercise, such as walking and running, helps strengthen your bones as you grow older, which will help prevent osteoporosis. The "Nurses Health Study" found that the women who walked for at least four hours a week at a moderate pace had a 41 percent lower risk of hip fracture than sedentary women who walked for less than an hour a week. Walking eight hours a week was associated with a 58 percent lower risk of hip fractures.

The great thing about walking is that almost anyone can do it, and it fits into your schedule easily. All you need is a good pair of walking shoes. And if you've got a walking buddy or two, you can socialize while you walk—the time flies by. If you don't have a buddy, invest in a portable CD player and headphones, and you can listen to whatever music or motivational CD inspires you.

What About Strength Training?

Studies have shown that women who take part in regular strength training will have better bone density after menopause as well. So put the two together—weight-bearing exercise plus strength training—and you've got it made. What are we waiting for?

Got Good-Tasting Dairy Products?

There are several great reasons to lower the fat in dairy products. A good portion of the fat in dairy is saturated fat, so as dairy companies skim the fat off, so to speak, they will also decrease the amount of saturated fat, cholesterol, and calories. Generally, when the fat is removed from dairy products, the protein and calcium portion is increased.

Great-Tasting Reduced-Fat Cheeses

The cheeses with only a little fat taken out, like Cracker Barrel Light Sharp Cheddar with 6 grams of fat per ounce, are more likely to look and taste like regular cheese, because they still have a respectable amount of fat. I've been using reduced-fat cheeses for years and have found that they work great in every situation that calls for cheese (in recipes, on crackers, for grilled cheese sandwiches, etc.) Fat-free cheeses just aren't going to compare to regular cheese, because they have zero fat per ounce, whereas regular cheese has about 9 grams of fat per ounce. They aren't going to taste or melt like the cheese we know and love.

BONE-FRIENDLY WORKOUT TIPS

- Do strengthening exercises for 30 minutes, two to three days a week and include moves to benefit the back and hips, such as Curves or weight machines.
- Aim for 30 minutes of weight-bearing aerobic exercise at least three or more days a week. Try to work in some really fun weight-bearing types of exercises once in a while, too, like hiking or dancing.
- If you have been diagnosed with bone loss or are over sixty years young, get a medical evaluation before you start weight training or any regular exercise program.
- Supplement your new exercise attitude with a calcium- and vitamin-D-rich eating plan (1,200–1,500 mg of calcium and 400–600 IU of vitamin D per day).

---

10 Recipes to Boost Your Bones

Berry Crepes with Yogurt Cream

You can quickly whip up this crepe batter using a blender. If you have crepes leftover, you can freeze them in a resealable bag. For the berry filling, you can use whatever berries you like, or mix it up with several types of berries, such as boysenberries and sliced strawberries.

Makes about 10–12 crepes • Serving Size: 1 crepe

CREPES:

2 large eggs

½ cup egg substitute

1 tablespoon canola oil

½ cup white or cake flour

½ cup whole-wheat pastry flour

½ teaspoon salt

1 teaspoon vanilla extract

FILLING:

About 4 cups of fresh berries, washed and drained (if using strawberries, remove green tops and slice)

¼ cup ground flaxseeds (optional)

3 tablespoons liqueur, such as Grand Marnier (optional)

1½ cups lowfat vanilla yogurt

1. Add all the crepe ingredients to a blender (eggs, egg substitute, canola oil, flours, salt, vanilla extract) and pulse until batter is smooth. Scrape down sides of blender with spatula and briefly blend.
2. Heat a 10-inch nonstick frying pan over medium heat. Spray bottom lightly with canola oil cooking spray. Pour ¼ cup of batter into pan, tilting pan to coat bottom completely with batter. It should be in a shape of a circle.
3. Cook about 1 minute per side or until golden brown. Remove crepe to serving plate and repeat with remaining batter.

4. In a medium bowl, toss the fruit with flaxseeds and powdered sugar and liqueur, if desired.

5. Add about ⅓ cup of fruit down the center of each crepe and top with a spoonful of vanilla yogurt. Roll up crepe around the filling.

Nutritional Facts *(1 crepe) if 10 crepes per recipe and if using raspberries and blackberries in the filling*: 134 calories, 6.5 g protein, 21 g carbohydrate, 3 g fat (0.8 g saturated fat, 1.5 g monounsaturated fat, 0.7 g polyunsaturated fat, 0.3 g omega-3 fatty acids, 0.4 g omega-6 fatty acids), 44 mg cholesterol, 3.5 g fiber, 164 mg sodium. Calories from fat: 21 percent.

32 RE vitamin A, 12 mg vitamin C, 29 IU vitamin D, 1.6 IU vitamin E, 0.3 mcg vitamin B$_{12}$, 46 mcg folate, 95 mg calcium, 11 mcg selenium.

Weight Watchers POINTS = 2 points

Best Spinach Dip

This is a light, high-calcium rendition of that colorful and tasty party staple—spinach dip. It's the fat-free sour cream, tofu, and the frozen spinach that contribute the calcium, and the spinach and tofu also add a boost of magnesium. You can make the dip and carve out a sourdough round (cutting the carved-out bread into bite-size cubes) a day ahead of time. Keep the bread in extra-large resealable bags, and store the dip, covered, in the refrigerator. Then fill the sourdough serving bowl just before the party. You can also enjoy this dip with cut vegetables or high-fiber, whole-grain crackers. *Makes about 8 servings • Serving size: ½ cup*

1 cup light silken tofu (the package should say "for use in smoothies")

1¾ cups fat-free or light sour cream

1 tablespoon mayonnaise

1 1.8-ounce box dry leek soup mix or vegetable soup mix

1 cup jicama, finely chopped (1 4-ounce can water chestnuts, drained and chopped, can be used)

10 ounces frozen chopped spinach, thawed, drained, excess water squeezed out

1. In mixing bowl, on medium speed, beat together tofu, sour cream, mayonnaise, and soup mix until smooth and well blended.

2. Stir in the jicama and chopped spinach. Cover bowl and chill in the refrigerator 6 hours or overnight.

3. When ready to serve, if serving in a bread bowl, remove top and interior of sourdough bread round, making a bowl. Fill the bread bowl with the spinach mixture. Cut the carved-out bread top into bite-size cubes for dipping. Serve the spinach dip–filled bread bowl with the bread cubes.

Nutritional Facts (*per serving*): 121 calories, 6 g protein, 17 g carbohydrate, 3.5 g fat (1.2 g saturated fat, 0.9 g monounsaturated fat, 0.9 g polyunsaturated fat, 0.4 g omega-3 fatty acids, 0.4 g omega-6 fatty acids), 7 mg cholesterol, 2.2 g fiber, 590 mg sodium. Calories from fat: 26 percent.

370 RE vitamin A, 14 mg vitamin C, 0 IU vitamin D, 7 IU vitamin E, 0.2 mcg vitamin B_{12}, 49 mcg folate, 143 mg calcium, 0.5 mcg selenium.

Vegetable Soufflé Squares

There is so much more going on in this dish than zucchini—but I barely noticed the zucchini with the artichoke-heart chunks and chopped onion and garlic mixed throughout. This is one of those appetizers (or breakfasts) that you can make ahead of time, keep in the refrigerator, and then reheat (or not) when you are ready to eat it.

Makes 8 appetizer servings or 4 entrée servings • Serving size: 2" x 4" piece

1 6-ounce jar of marinated artichoke hearts

1½ teaspoons canola oil

1 small white or yellow onion, chopped

1 teaspoon garlic, minced

2 cups diced firm tofu, drained well

1 cup zucchini, grated (approximately 1 regular-size zucchini)

2 large eggs

½ cup egg substitute (or 4 egg whites)

¼ cup plain bread crumbs (seasoned bread crumbs can be used)

½ teaspoon dried oregano

½ teaspoon salt

¼ teaspoon ground pepper, or to taste

½–1 teaspoon Tabasco, or to taste

1½ cups shredded reduced-fat sharp cheddar cheese

2 tablespoons fresh parsley, chopped (or 2 teaspoons dried parsley flakes)

1. Preheat oven to 325 degrees. Spray a 8x8-inch (or 9x9-inch) baking dish with canola oil cooking spray.
2. Open artichoke hearts and empty into a colander. Rinse well and drain. Cut larger pieces into small chunks; set aside.

3. Add canola oil to a medium nonstick frying pan and heat over medium heat. Add onion, garlic, and tofu, and sauté for 3–5 minutes. Stir in artichoke heart pieces and grated zucchini and stir well. Remove from heat and set aside.

4. In a large mixing bowl, add eggs, egg substitute, bread crumbs, oregano, salt, pepper, and Tabasco. Beat on low until well blended. Stir in cheese, parsley, and artichoke heart mixture.

5. Pour mixture into prepared baking pan. Bake for 30 minutes or until egg batter is firm. Let sit 5–10 minutes and cut into small appetizer-size square servings or larger entrée servings. Serve hot or cold.

Nutritional Facts (*per appetizer serving*): 188 calories, 16 g protein, 12 g carbohydrate, 8.5 g fat (3.2 g saturated fat, 2.7 g monounsaturated fat, 2.2 g polyunsaturated fat, 0.3 g omega-3 fatty acids, 1.9 g omega-6 fatty acids), 64 mg cholesterol, 2.5 g fiber, 469 mg sodium. Calories from fat: 40 percent.

102 RE vitamin A, 10 mg vitamin C, 11 IU vitamin D, 1.1 IU vitamin E, 0.5 mcg vitamin B$_{12}$, 53 mcg folate, 289 mg calcium, 10 mcg selenium.

Easy Crustless Broccoli Quiche

This quiche's featured ingredient, broccoli, contributes calcium and some magnesium. The eggs and milk add vitamin D, and the cheese gives the calcium a big boost. We save calories and fat grams here by skipping the pastry crust, switching to reduced-fat cheese, and using half real eggs and half egg substitute.   *Makes 4 servings • Serving size: one-quarter of a 9" pie*

2 tablespoons Parmesan cheese,
    shredded or grated
2 tablespoons unseasoned dry
    bread crumbs
2 large eggs
¼ cup egg substitute or 2 egg whites
1½ cups fat-free half-and-half (whole milk
    can be substituted)
¼ teaspoon salt (optional)

½ teaspoon garlic powder
½ teaspoon onion powder (¼ cup finely
    chopped onion can be substituted)
¼ teaspoon Tabasco
4 ounces reduced-fat sharp cheddar cheese,
    shredded (about 1 cup)
1½ cups broccoli florets, steamed or
    microwaved until just tender,
    and diced

1. Preheat oven to 350 degrees. Coat the inside of a 9-inch-deep pie plate with canola oil cooking spray. Mix Parmesan and bread crumbs together in a small bowl, then pour into the prepared pie plate and tilt it around to coat the inside of the plate with the mixture.

2. In a mixing bowl, beat the eggs, egg substitute, half-and-half, salt (if desired), garlic powder, onion powder, and Tabasco together on medium speed until smooth.

3. Sprinkle cheese and broccoli evenly into the bottom of the prepared pie plate.

4. Pour egg mixture into the pie plate and gently stir mixture lightly with a fork to mix the ingredients together.

5. Place in the oven and bake for 40–45 minutes, until the edges are browned and puffy and the center is set.

Nutritional Facts *(per serving)*: 251 calories, 22 g protein, 18 g carbohydrate, 9.8 g fat (5 g saturated fat, 1.2 g monounsaturated fat, 0.5 g polyunsaturated fat, 0.1 g omega-3 fatty acids, 0.4 g omega-6 fatty acids), 132 mg cholesterol, 2 g fiber, 503 mg sodium. Calories from fat: 35 percent.

326 RE vitamin A, 47 mg vitamin C, 95 IU vitamin D, 1.2 IU vitamin E, 0.7 mcg vitamin B_{12}, 64 mcg folate, 563 mg calcium, 11 mcg selenium.

Heavenly (Lightened) Crab-Stuffed Deviled Eggs

This recipe will give you some vitamin D from the egg yolks, and the crab will contribute calcium and magnesium. In order to lighten this up, I use half the yolks and blend them with 2 teaspoons mayonnaise and 3 tablespoons fat-free sour cream instead of using all mayonnaise.

Makes 4 servings • Serving size: 2 halves

8 large eggs, hard-boiled, peeled, and cut
   in half lengthwise

3 tablespoons fat-free sour cream

2 teaspoons mayonnaise

2 teaspoons fresh tarragon, finely chopped
   (¾ teaspoon dried tarragon can
   be used)

1 tablespoon shallots, minced

1 teaspoon lemon juice (increase to 2
   teaspoons if desired)

2 pinches (or more) cayenne pepper

¼ teaspoon Tabasco

¾ cup (about 4 ounces) cooked crabmeat,
   shredded and shells removed

Salt and pepper to taste (optional)

Paprika (optional)

Tarragon sprig (optional)

1. Scoop out egg yolks and throw half of them away. Place remaining yolks in a medium bowl. Mash with fork and mix in sour cream, mayonnaise, tarragon, shallots, lemon juice, cayenne, and Tabasco. Or you can beat in a small mixing bowl if you prefer. Stir in the crabmeat. Season to taste with salt and pepper.

2. Carefully spoon the crab mixture into the cavity of each egg-white half, about 1 heaping tablespoon for each. Cover and refrigerate until ready to serve. Garnish each egg with a sprinkle of paprika and a small tarragon sprig if desired.

Nutritional Facts *(per serving)*: 145 calories, 15 g protein, 3.5 g carbohydrate, 7.5 g fat (2 g saturated fat, 2.5 g monounsaturated fat, 1.9 g polyunsaturated fat, 0.2 g omega-3 fatty acids, 0.7 g omega-6 fatty acids), 237 mg cholesterol, 0 g fiber, 202 mg sodium. Calories from fat: 46 percent.

123 RE vitamin A, 2 mg vitamin C, 26 IU vitamin D, 1.2 IU vitamin E, 2.2 mcg vitamin B$_{12}$, 32 mcg folate, 68 mg calcium, 28 mcg selenium.

Homemade Frozen Fruit Sorbet

This is a fun way to enjoy your high-calcium lowfat yogurt. You can add a packet of Splenda if you like, but to me it tastes great without it. The flaxseeds will add some magnesium and fiber, as well as some phytoestrogens and omega-3s, into the picture.

Makes 1 serving • Serving size: 1¼ cup

6 ounces lowfat vanilla yogurt

⅔ cup frozen boysenberries (or other frozen berries or peaches)

1 packet Splenda (optional)

1 tablespoon ground flaxseeds

1. Add yogurt, boysenberries, and Splenda (if desired) to the blender or food processor and pulse until a nice mixture is made.
2. Add to a serving dish and stir in flaxseeds.

Nutritional Facts (*per serving*): 229 calories, 11 g protein, 37 g carbohydrate, 5 g fat (1.6 g saturated fat, 1.2 g monounsaturated fat, 2 g polyunsaturated fat, 1.5 g omega-3 fatty acids, 0.5 g omega-6 fatty acids), 8 mg cholesterol, 6 g fiber, 116 mg sodium. Calories from fat: 20 percent.

28 RE vitamin A, 5 mg vitamin C, 3 IU vitamin D, 1.3 IU vitamin E, 1 mcg vitamin B_{12}, 97 mcg folate, 331 mg calcium, 9.3 mcg selenium.

Orange-Strawberry-Banana Freeze

This reminds me of the frothy drinks that the Orange Julius chain makes. This drink went over big with a crowd of teenagers that were visiting my house while I was making it—it's always a good sign if the teens like it. The calcium in this drink comes from the calcium-fortified orange juice and calcium- and vitamin-D-fortified vanilla soymilk. This recipe calls for a blender, but a food processor will also work. *Makes 2 large drinks • Serving size: 2½ cups*

½ cup orange juice (if you use calcium-
  fortified orange juice, add the extra
  calcium to the nutrition analysis
  below)
¼ cup egg substitute (it's pasteurized, so
  there is no risk of salmonella
  poisoning)
2 tablespoons sugar
½ cup vanilla soymilk (I like the Silk
  brand)

½ teaspoon coconut extract
¼ teaspoon almond extract
2 medium ripe bananas, peeled
2 heaping cups (about 7 ounces)
  of frozen strawberries, unsweetened,
  slightly thawed
3 cups ice

1. Add all the ingredients to a blender, in the order listed above, and let sit a few minutes
   to dissolve the sugar.
2. Blend on medium speed for about 15 seconds or until the ice is crushed and the drink
   is well blended. Pour into 2 large 8-ounce glasses. Drink through a straw if desired.

Nutritional Facts (*per serving*): 276 calories, 7 g protein, 63 g carbohydrate, 1.7 g fat (0.3 g saturated fat, 0.1 g monounsaturated fat, 0.2 g polyunsaturated fat, 0.2 g omega-3 fatty acids, 0.5 g omega-6 fatty acids), 0 mg cholesterol, 5.5 g fiber, 90 mg sodium. Calories from fat: 5.5 percent.

82 RE vitamin A, 84 mg vitamin C, 38 IU vitamin D, 1.6 IU vitamin E, 1.1 mcg vitamin B_{12}, 83 mcg folate, 116 mg calcium, 2.3 mcg selenium.

Quick Vanilla or Chocolate Pudding

I like using the sugar-free instant pudding, but you can use the regular sugar-sweetened pudding mix if you prefer. I include nutrition analyses for both below. Imagine my surprise when I learned that instant pudding doesn't "set" when using soymilk. I'm sure there's a food science explanation. But, being the stubborn dietitian that I am, I tried half vanilla soymilk and half lowfat milk, and voilà!

Makes 4 servings • Serving size: ½ cup

1 cup cold vanilla soymilk
1 cup cold 1 percent lowfat milk (2 percent
  or whole can also be used)

1 1.4-ounce box Jell-O Brand Fat Free Sugar
  Free Instant Reduced Calorie Pudding
  and Pie Filling—Vanilla or Chocolate

1. Add cold soymilk and milk to a large mixing bowl. Sprinkle pudding mix evenly over the top.
2. With mixer, beat pudding mixture together on medium-low speed for 2 minutes, stopping to scrape the sides of the bowl a couple times.
3. Once mixed well, pour at once into 4 serving dishes or cups. Cover each serving and refrigerate. Pudding will be soft-set and ready to eat within 15 minutes. When covered, the pudding will keep well for two to three days.

Note: Sugar-free pudding mix contains aspartame and acesulfame potassium (sweeteners). Each serving also contains 5–9 milligrams of isoflavones, 1.5 grams of soy protein, and about 15 percent of the Daily Value for vitamin D and calcium.

Nutritional Facts (*per serving*): 58 calories, 4 g protein, 7 g carbohydrate, 1.5 g fat (0.4 g saturated fat, 0.2 g monounsaturated fat, 0 g polyunsaturated fat, 0 g omega-3 fatty acids, 0 g omega-6 fatty acids), 4 mg cholesterol, 0 g fiber, 85 mg sodium. Calories from fat: 23 percent.

50 RE vitamin A, 0 mg vitamin C, 55 IU vitamin D, 0.8 mcg vitamin B_{12}, 6 mcg folate, 143 mg calcium.

Strawberries-and-Cream Smoothie

You can enjoy this smoothie using a spoon or a straw—it's delicious. You can stir in a tablespoon of ground flaxseeds, too, if you want. You'll need a blender or food processor for this recipe.   *Makes 1 smoothie • Serving size: 2 cups*

½ cup light cherry-vanilla yogurt
1 cup sliced strawberries
½ cup light vanilla ice cream or
  lowfat frozen yogurt

1 tablespoon ground flaxseeds (optional)
1 cup ice cubes (optional)

1. Add all the ingredients to a blender or small food processor and pulse until smooth and completely blended.
2. Pour into 1 8-ounce glass and enjoy.

Nutritional Facts *(per serving)*: 217 calories, 9 g protein, 36 g carbohydrate, 5.5 g fat (1.7 g saturated fat, 1.3 g monounsaturated fat, 2.2 g polyunsaturated fat, 1.6 g omega-3 fatty acids, 0.6 g omega-6 fatty acids), 12 mg cholesterol, 6 g fiber, 101 mg sodium. Calories from fat: 23 percent.

27 RE vitamin A, 96 mg vitamin C, 0.3 IU vitamin D, 1.1 IU vitamin E, 0.2 mcg vitamin B_{12}, 55 mcg folate, 285 mg calcium, 2.6 mcg selenium.

Yogurt Parfait

Yogurt is at the very top of the calcium food list, so I know you want to eat more of it. But let's face it, yogurt can get a little bit boring when it's straight from the container day after day. But here's a fun way to eat your yogurt—in fact, it might even pass for dessert.

Makes 2 servings • Serving size: 2 cups

2 cups vanilla-flavored light or lowfat yogurt
2 cups sliced strawberries, (frozen strawberries may also be used)

2 heaping tablespoons fresh or frozen blueberries, slightly thawed
½ cup reduced-fat granola

1. Spoon ½ cup yogurt into dessert cup or 8-inch-tall glass.
2. Top yogurt with ½ cup strawberries, followed by a heaping tablespoon of blueberries.
3. Spread remaining yogurt over the blueberries and top with granola.

Nutritional Facts *(per serving)*: 256 calories, 10 g protein, 51.5 g carbohydrate, 1.7 g fat (0.4 g saturated fat, 0.4 g monounsaturated fat, 0.8 g polyunsaturated fat, 0.2 g omega-3 fatty acids, 0.6 g omega-6 fatty acids), 5 mg cholesterol, 6 g fiber, 180 mg sodium. Calories from fat: 6 percent.

85 RE vitamin A, 100 mg vitamin C, 17 IU vitamin D, 3.7 IU vitamin E, 0.5 mcg vitamin B_{12}, 73 mcg folate, 384 mg calcium, 5 mcg selenium.

10.

How to Reduce Your Risk of Colon Cancer Without HRT

Somehow the description "uncontrolled reproduction of abnormal cells" doesn't sound as frightening as the word it describes: cancer. This six-letter word single-handedly sends shockwaves through men and women, myself included. But there are many reasons for being more hopeful and less fearful today than in the past.

Scientists have been gaining a better understanding of the many causes of cancer and the complex process that causes cancer cells to grow. And the more we know about the initiation and growth of cancer, the better our chances are at preventing it altogether. And prevent it we can; scientists estimate that approximately 30 to 40 percent of all cancers are linked to diet and related lifestyle factors. Granted, there are no guarantees with eating and living healthy, but it does tip the scales in your favor.

If you think you have to pop a handful of supplements to keep yourself on the anticancer track, think again. Cancer research keeps pointing us in the direction of food, not supplements; clinical trials have not yet been able to demonstrate the same protective effects from taking supplements as you get from food.

Here's a little heads-up, though. Many of the food suggestions below will point you unmistakably in the direction of your produce section, which is filled with high-nutrient, colorful fruits and vegetables. Studies, both epidemiological and experimental, continue to indicate that people who consume large amounts of fruits and vegetables have a lower risk of cancer.

CANCER STATS

- About 1.2 million Americans are diagnosed with cancer each year.
- Breast cancer is the most common cancer among American women.
- Breast cancer and prostate cancer are the most common cancers in the United States (excluding non-melanoma skin cancer), followed by lung, colon, and bladder cancer.
- If everyone ate at least five or more servings of vegetables and fruits per day, cancer rates could fall by as much as 20 percent, according to the American Institute for Cancer Research.
- If you ate a pound of fruits and vegetables each day, evidence suggests you would significantly lower your risk of lung, esophageal, and stomach cancer.
- DNA (the set of genetic instructions that tells your body's cells how to reproduce and grow) takes little "punches" over the years, possibly eventually damaging it to the point where the normal cell-growth process is replaced by uncontrolled abnormal cell growth. We can avoid many of these everyday punches, such as exposure to tobacco, alcohol, and the sun's UV rays, and eating a diet that lacks important nutrients.

Third on the List: Colon Cancer

Colon cancer is the third most common cancer among American women, and it becomes more common with age, usually striking women over age fifty. As our age increases, our risk of developing colon cancer quickly increases, too. Add on an additional increased risk if one of your family members has had colon cancer.

One of the health benefits of being on HRT during and after menopause is a reduced incidence of colon cancer. But HRT isn't the only way to reduce your risk of colon cancer through menopause and beyond. There are lots of good dietary habits that will decrease that risk as well.

The Diet and Lifestyle Laundry List

You can do eight specific things to help prevent colon cancer, according to the Harvard Center for Cancer Prevention's "your cancer risk" website, www.yourcancerrisk.harvard.edu

- **Get regular screening tests starting at age fifty.** (If you have a family history of colon cancer, then you may want to get screened sooner.) Although screenings for cancer are not specifically able to prevent the cancer, early detection is the key factor in a positive outcome—not just preventing death but preventing serious complications and compromised well-being. And precancerous polyps can be found and removed.
- **Eat less red meat.** Eating less than three servings of red meat a week will help lower your risk of colon cancer.
- **Take a multivitamin with folic acid every day.** Taking a multivitamin with folic acid every day can help lower your risk of colon cancer. You can also eat folate-rich plant foods every day; some evidence suggests that the folate found in fruits, vegetables, whole grains, and beans may be linked to the prevention of colon cancer.
- **Eat more vegetables.** Eating three or more servings of vegetables a day will help lower your risk of colon, breast, and lung cancer. Vegetable consumption has been shown to have the strongest and most consistent association with colon cancer risk reduction. Recent data suggest that fruits are protective but probably not as protective against colon cancer as vegetables.
- **Maintain a healthy weight.** Avoid obesity, especially abdominal obesity. Twenty percent of all cancer deaths in women are associated with being overweight or obese, according to a new study from the American Cancer Society. Researchers have already found that breast and colorectal cancers are linked to excess body weight, but this study identified other cancers as well (stomach, prostate, cervical, ovarian, liver, and pancreatic cancer).
- **Limit the amount of alcohol you drink.**
- **Be physically active for at least 30 minutes every day.**
- **Take an aspirin every day.** (But be sure to check with your doctor first.)

Certain vegetables do seem to offer us more protection against colon cancer than others, presumably because they are rich sources of various anticancer phytochemicals, vitamins, or minerals. The recipes in this chapter not only aim to help you to up the amount of vegetables in your diet, but also to work some of the veggie powerhouses into your day.

Powerful Phytochemicals and Nutrients

You can probably already tell that when it comes to cancer and diet recommendations, there are some foods and beverages we need to eat more of and some foods and beverages we need to eat less of. We'll start with the foods we need to eat more of, and work our way down to the diet items we desperately need to moderate.

General Cancer-Prevention Properties

NCI (National Cancer Institute) scientists singled out these six foods as deserving of special study because they show potential cancer-fighting abilities: flaxseed, garlic, licorice root, vegetables from the parsnip family, citrus fruits, and soybeans. Critical nutrients and phytochemicals with their food sources are listed below.

FLAVONOIDS

Flavonoids are a family of anticancer phytochemicals found in all sorts of plant foods, including citrus fruits, blueberries, cranberries, cherries, and apples. Beans, nuts, olive oil, broccoli, onions, celery hearts, rutabagas, tea, and red wine also contain flavonoids. They act as antioxidants and seem to help protect us at the beginning and promotional stages of cancer. (The second phase of the cancer process is called the *promotional phase,* because cancer has been initiated and the cells now must divide for cancer to occur.)

Prevention qualities specific to colon cancer

LIGNANS

Lignans are phyto- or plant estrogens that appear to be beneficial throughout the promotional phase of carcinogenesis, potentially reducing the risk of certain kinds of cancer. Although flaxseed is the richest food source of lignans, barley, buckwheat, millet, oats, broccoli, carrots, cauliflower, spinach, and legumes (including soybeans) also contain lignans. Flaxseed has been shown over the short term to decrease some early markers of colon cancer risk, according to flaxseed researchers at the University of Toronto.

QUERCETIN

Onions are rich in the substance *quercetin* (23 mg quercetin per 100 grams), which is a flavonoid phytochemical thought to have antioxidative and anticarcinogenic properties. Studies on rats demonstrated an inhibition of induced colon tumors when their diet contained quercetin. Cranberries (14 milligrams quercetin per 100 grams) and broccoli (3 mg per 100 grams) contain smaller amounts of quercetin.

TOMATOES AND TOMATO PRODUCTS

Tomatoes contain the anticancer standout *lycopene,* a potent antioxidant that is also found in other fruits such as pink grapefruit and watermelon. Recent studies show that lycopene may help protect against breast, colon, lung, and prostate cancer. When looking for foods that contain lycopene, there are two rules to follow: (1) raw is not best—cooked or processed tomato products actually contain more lycopene, and (2) a little fat, such as olive oil, in a recipe makes lycopene more available to body tissues.

FOLATE (FOLIC ACID)

What do spinach, beans, orange juice, and strawberries have in common? They are all rich in folate, a vitamin that cancer scientists believe may be essential to the body's effort to prevent cancer in two ways:

1. Folate helps make two basic building blocks of DNA. As long as there is enough folate in our diet, the body is able to assemble DNA in the normal way.
2. Folate also seems to assist in *methylation* (a process in which single atoms of carbon are added to other molecules so important reactions can happen).

Even diets that are low in fat and high in fiber are associated with colon cancer risk, if they are deficient in folic acid. The results of a recent Dutch study showed that the higher your daily intake of folate from food, the lower your risk of colon cancer. It doesn't get much simpler than that! How about practically eliminating the risk of colon cancer? In a recent study of women called the Nurses Health Study, a diet high in folate (400 mcg/day) appeared to virtually eliminate the risk of colon cancer in women whose diets were initially low in folate and who had a family history of colorectal cancer.

Fill Up with Fiber

If you eat a high-fat, low-fiber diet, your risk for colon cancer increases, according to the American Cancer Society. Fiber may reduce the risk of colon cancer in four different ways:

1. The fermentation of fiber in the colon may produce *butyrate,* a by-product that has anticarcinogenic effects (American Institute for Cancer Research).
2. Fiber is one of the bioactive, potentially anticancer components in citrus fruits and other high-nutrient fruits, vegetables, beans, and whole grains.
3. Fiber may also be chemoprotective (protective against cancer progression), due to its influence on sex hormone levels, possibly decreasing the risk of hormone-dependent cancers.
4. When you eat a diet that is naturally rich in fiber (because you are choosing fruits and vegetables, whole grains, and beans), your diet is also usually rich in micronutrients and nonnutritive ingredients that have additional health benefits.

Source: *JADA* 2002 Jul; 102(7): 993–1000, "Position of the ADA: Health Implications of Dietary Fiber").

Fishing for Answers

It's a great goal for a plethora of health reasons to eat fish two or three times a week; and we might be able to add a reduced risk of colon cancer to the list of reasons. When you eat more fish, you are more likely to eat less red meat, which may also help the colon. But the main reason is that omega-3 fats found in fish have been shown, in animal studies, to slow or prevent the growth of certain cancers. There is still a lot of research needed in this area, but there have been some studies suggesting that omega-3s may reduce the risk of colon cancer.

Whole Grains and Beans

It's time to trade your white rice for brown, your French bread for whole-wheat, and your sugary cereal for a bowl of oatmeal to reduce your risk of cancer. When we eat whole grains, along with a nice dose of fiber, we also get phytochemicals with anticarcinogenic properties. *Saponins* in whole grains, beans, and soy, for example, may neutralize cancer-causing substances in the intestines and possibly reduce the risk of colon cancer (American Institute for Cancer Research). *Phytic Acid,* a phytochemical in whole-wheat products, may suppress the oxygen-related reactions in the colon that produce damaging free radicals—unstable molecules that damage cells and are believed to contribute to the development of many age-related diseases, including cancer.

Too Much of a Good Thing

So far, we've been discussing foods and food components that we need more of because they may help protect our bodies from colon cancer. The flip side to that story is the foods or substances that possibly increase our risk because we consume too much of them in the typical American diet. These food suggestions are usually the toughest to swallow, but ideally we want to do both—eat more protective foods and eat less of the foods and beverages that may be increasing our risk of cancer. Are you ready for the "too much" list? Here we go!

1. **Too many calories:** Eating too many calories is suspected to be one of the major contributors to the high rates of colon cancer in Western countries.

2. **Insulin resistance:** When we eat more calories than we need, our body stores the extra calories as body fat. As this excess body fat deposits around the stomach and as the excess weight reaches obese amounts, we become more at risk for diabetes and insulin resistance (a situation when your body cells don't respond to the insulin that is circulating in your system). Unfortunately, insulin resistance may be linked to colon cancer, although research has not yet definitively made this link.

    Recent evidence indicates that chronic hyperinsulinemia (high levels of insulin circulating in the bloodstream) may increase the risk of colon cancer. Insulin resistance and the hyperinsulinemia that results from it are thought to be brought about in part by excessive calories (energy), as well as other aspects of a typical American diet, with high levels of saturated fat and refined or processed carbohydrates.

3. **Too much sugar:** A high-sugar diet directly or indirectly increases the frequency of permanent change or transformation of body cells in the colons of laboratory rats—and as the amount of sugar goes up, the amount of mutations go up, too, according to a Danish study. Coincidentally, both sugar intake and colon cancer rates are high in the Western world; these study results call for an examination of a possible direct relationship between the two.

Here's the Beef

Reviews of the literature on colon cancer suggest that while a high-protein diet doesn't seem to increase the risk of colon cancer, a diet high in meat might. Following along these lines, a recent Japanese study concluded that as consumption of *animal* protein and fats increased, incidence of colorectal cancer increased as well, but colorectal cancer incidence decreased as consumption of plant protein increased, along with amounts of carbohydrate and cereal grains.

Uruguay and Argentina have two of the highest rates of breast and colon cancer in the world—people in those countries also eat more beef than people in most other countries around the world. Coincidence? Consumption of red meat and the heterocyclic amines (HCAs) that sometimes go with it has been associated with an increased risk of colorectal cancer.

SEVEN THINGS YOU CAN DO TO HAVE YOUR GRILLED MEAT AND EAT IT, TOO

1. Trim visible fat from meat before marinating and grilling.
2. Eat your grilled meat with fruits and vegetables that are rich in antioxidants, such as vitamin C and beta-carotene.
3. Precook meat for a few minutes in a microwave oven before putting it on the grill. Not only does this cut down on the time the meat has to be on the grill, it also removes some of the juices, which in turn reduces the amount of HCAs that can be produced.
4. Don't grill every day—keep it as an occasional or weekly treat.

HIGH HEAT PRODUCES HCAs

Cooking meat on the grill has been implicated in creating cancer-causing agents, largely because of heterocyclic amines (HCAs). HCAs cause genetic mutations (permanent changes) in cells and form when high heat is applied to a combination of amino acids (mainly creatine found in the blood and muscle of animals, which includes beef, pork, fowl, and lamb). So far, we know that HCAs cause tumors in animals and they are most often associated with cancer of the gastrointestinal tract. But this doesn't let animal fat off the hook—HCAs are also suspected of working together with fat to promote cancer growth.

5. Don't overcook your meat. Generally, the more well done the meat, the more HCAs it contains. (This is a hard one for those of us, like me, who like our meat well done—the blacker, the better.)

6. And the marinade shall set you free! New studies suggest that marinating your meat or poultry at least three minutes before cooking may lower HCA formation by 94 to 96 percent.

7. Choose marinades that are low in oil to minimize fat dripping onto the coals and causing high flames.

Processed Meats

In the 1970s, scientists detected carcinogenic compounds known as *nitrosamines* in many favorite processed meats, such as bacon, sausage, cured pork, dried beef, and hot dogs. Out of all of them, bacon had one of the highest levels. Nitrosamines are formed during the breakdown of nitrites and nitrates, which are what is used to cure and preserve meat, give it that pink look, and protect against botulism.

There is some evidence that processed (nitrite-preserved) meat is linked to colon cancer, although it is possible that people who eat processed meat also eat less fiber, adding to their increased risk. It is a good idea, though, to reduce your intake of nitrite-preserved meat, such as hot dogs, ham, corned beef, bacon, bratwurst, salami, etc.

However, there is a way to actually decrease the formation of nitrosamines from nitrates and nitrites: adding antioxidants to the product, such as ascorbic acid, ascorbate, vitamin C and tocopherol, or vitamin E, or adding P-coumaric and chlorogenic acids (phytochemicals found in fruits and vegetables). Many manufacturers are already adding these to their prod-

HCAs AND BREAST CANCER

If you prefer your burger burned and your milk whole, you may be increasing your risk of breast cancer. HCAs may play a role in the formation of premenopausal breast cancer. They are found in the fat component of dairy products and are formed in well-done meat. The Iowa Women's Health Study reported that women who regularly ate well-done meat had higher risks of breast cancer compared to women with high intakes of less well-done meat.

ucts (check the labels), but you can also eat your preserved meat with some fruits and vegetables that are naturally high in vitamin C!

Too Much Alcohol

Alcohol may be promoting carcinogenesis by delaying DNA repair or disrupting DNA methylation. But limiting the amount of alcohol you drink to less than one or more servings a day can help lower your risk of breast and colon cancer (Harvard Center for Cancer Prevention) and possibly other cancers as well. Eating the recommended daily intake of folate seems to be vital for women at higher risk of developing breast cancer due to imbibing alcohol—even at the level of one drink a day (Researchers from Brigham and Women's Hospital and Harvard Medical School, Boston).

Use It or Lose It!

Exercise may decrease the production of the same hormones and growth factors that fat cells secrete, which help promote cancer. For example, new evidence links exercise with a 40 to 50 percent reduction in colon cancer risk. Exercise may work its magic by speeding the movement of food through the intestines and decreasing bile acid secretion.

Inactivity, excess body weight, and carrying excess weight around your middle are all consistent risk factors for colon cancer. If you stay active and exercise as much as possible, you will:

1. Speed the passage of stools through the intestines, which should help reduce your risk of colon cancer.
2. Help reduce excess weight, which can increase your risk of colon cancer.
3. Reduce your risk of colon cancer. Since 1980, seven out of eight studies examining the relationship between exercise and colon cancer found that exercise does reduce the risk.

4. Cut colon cancer risk by 10 percent. Just 30 minutes of walking a day can cut colon cancer risk by 10 percent, according to the Harvard Nurse's study. A Swedish study found that a sedentary job was associated with a 30 percent increase in cancer risk—and most of us have sedentary jobs!

Recipes to Reduce the Risk of Colon Cancer

Easy Antipasto

A fun and quick way to get your veggies as a snack or with your entrée is to dress lightly cooked vegetables, such as broccoli and cauliflower florets or green beans, and some fresh veggies, such as jicama strips and tomato quarters, with some bottled light Italian dressing.

Makes about 5 servings • Serving size: 1 cup

1 cup broccoli florets, lightly steamed or microwaved

1 cup cauliflower florets, lightly steamed or microwaved

1 cup green beans, lightly steamed or microwaved

1 cup jicama, peeled and cut into 2-inch strips

1 cup cherry tomatoes, halved, or 1 small tomato, quartered

5 tablespoons bottled light Italian dressing

1. Add assorted vegetables to a medium-size bowl. Drizzle with the dressing and toss to coat the vegetables well.
2. Cover bowl and chill in refrigerator until needed.
3. Toss well before serving.

Nutritional Facts *(per serving)*: 56 calories, 2 g protein, 8 g carbohydrate, 2.4 g fat (0.2 g saturated fat, 0 g monounsaturated fat, 0.1 g polyunsaturated fat, 0.1 g omega-3 fatty acids, 0.5 g omega-6 fatty acids), 1 mg cholesterol, 3 g fiber, 99 mg sodium. Calories from fat: 28 percent.

388 RE vitamin A, 39 mg vitamin C, 0 IU vitamin D, 3.3 IU vitamin E, 3.7 mcg vitamin B_{12}, 192 mcg folate, 170 mg calcium, 38 mcg selenium.

Cream of Vegetable Soup

This just may be the heartiest, tastiest, healthiest, and most filling cream soup you have ever tasted. If you want to bring the richness of the milk down a notch, you can substitute low-fat milk instead of whole—but I prefer a little added creaminess!

Makes 6 servings • Serving size: 2 cups

1 large onion, chopped

2 tablespoons canola oil

3 cloves garlic, minced or pressed

2 medium sweet potatoes, peeled and chopped

2 medium zucchini, chopped

2 bunches broccoli, chopped, stems removed (about 3 cups)

1 quart low-sodium vegetable or chicken broth

1 large or 2 small potatoes, peeled and shredded (1½ cups frozen shredded hash browns can be used to save time)

½ teaspoon celery seed

¼ teaspoon dill weed (optional)

¼ teaspoon curry powder (add more to taste)

½ teaspoon pepper (add more to taste)

1½ cups whole milk (fat-free half-and-half can also be used)

1. In large nonstick saucepan, sauté onion in canola oil over medium heat until transparent. Add garlic, sweet potatoes, zucchini, and broccoli, and sauté lightly for 5 more minutes or until just tender.

2. Stir in broth, cover, and simmer 5 minutes.

3. Add shredded potatoes, celery seed, dill weed if desired, curry powder, and pepper to taste. Cover saucepan and simmer 10 minutes.

4. Add the soup to a blender or large food processor in two batches and pulse until nicely blended. Return to large saucepan and stir in milk and heat through, about 2 minutes.

Nutritional Facts (*per serving*): 193 calories, 7.5 g protein, 25 g carbohydrate, 8 g fat (2.2 g saturated fat, 3.5 g monounsaturated fat, 1.6 g polyunsaturated fat, 0.5 g omega-3 fatty acids, 1 g omega-6 fatty acids), 11 mg cholesterol, 4 g fiber, 119 mg sodium. Calories from fat: 37 percent.

974 RE vitamin A, 53 mg vitamin C, 25 IU vitamin D, 3 IU vitamin E, 0.2 mcg vitamin B_{12}, 56 mcg folate, 129 mg calcium, 3 mcg selenium.

Ovo-Vegetarian Matzo Ball Soup

People either love matzo ball soup or hate it—clearly I'm a lover. This is a vegetarian version of the famed soup. Each serving is brimming with nutrient-rich vegetables.

Makes 6 servings • Serving size: 2 cups

MATZO BALLS:

1 tablespoon canola oil

2–3 tablespoons vegetable broth or chicken broth

1 egg

¼ cup egg substitute

¾ cup matzo meal

1 teaspoon salt or less (optional)

SOUP:

6 green onions (white and part of green), sliced on a diagonal or coarsely chopped

6 celery stalks, sliced (about 1 ¼ cups)

2 cups baby carrots (sliced carrots can be substituted)

1 10-ounce box frozen spinach leaves or 4 cups fresh spinach leaves, firmly packed

8 cups vegetable broth or chicken broth

1 teaspoon dried parsley flakes

½ teaspoon dried, ground sage

½ teaspoon dried summer savory

1. Start by making the matzo balls. Blend canola oil, broth, egg, and egg substitute together in a large mixing bowl. Add matzo meal and salt, if desired, and blend well. Mix till uniform. (Add an additional tablespoon of broth if needed.) Cover mixing bowl and refrigerate for 15 minutes.
2. In a large nonstick saucepan, combine onions, celery, carrots, spinach, broth, and spices.
3. Bring to a boil. Reduce flame to a high simmer.
4. Remove matzo mixture from the refrigerator. Form about a tablespoon of the mixture into a ball using the palms of your hands. Repeat with the remaining mixture. Drop the balls into the gently boiling soup. Add spinach, stir, cover pot, and cook 30–40 minutes.
5. Spoon into 6 large soup bowls.

Nutritional Facts *(per serving)*: 160 calories, 8.5 g protein, 25 g carbohydrate, 5 g fat (0.5 g saturated fat, 1.7 g monounsaturated fat, 0.9 g polyunsaturated fat, 0.3 g omega-3 fatty acids, 0.6 g omega-6 fatty acids), 35 mg cholesterol, 4 g fiber, 1,450 mg sodium. Calories from fat: 28 percent.

1433 RE vitamin A, 19 mg vitamin C, 7 IU vitamin D, 2.2 IU vitamin E, 0.2 mcg vitamin B12, 88 mcg folate, 93 mg calcium, 4 mcg selenium.

Power Minestrone

This is a nutrient-packed soup that even your kids or teens will love! This soup has everything: beans, phytochemical-rich tomatoes, carrots, onion, and garlic.

Makes 5 large dinner servings • Serving size: 2 cups

5 cups low-sodium vegetable or
    beef broth

3 carrots, diced

3 large outer celery stalks, sliced at a
    diagonal

1 onion, chopped

3 to 4 cloves garlic, minced or pressed

1 teaspoon dried basil, crushed

½ teaspoon dried oregano, crushed

¼ teaspoon pepper

1 15-ounce can red kidney beans (or great
    northern beans), drained and rinsed

1 15-ounce can Italian-style stewed
    tomatoes (or regular stewed tomatoes)

2 cups zucchini, halved lengthwise and
    sliced

½ cup tiny shell macaroni (or similar
    shaped pasta)

4 tablespoons Parmesan cheese, grated
    (optional)

1. In a large saucepan, combine broth, carrot, celery, onion, garlic, basil, oregano, and pepper. Bring to a boil; reduce heat. Cover; simmer for 15 minutes.

2. Stir in beans, tomatoes, zucchini, and macaroni. Return to boil; cover and reduce heat to simmer. Cook 10 minutes more or until vegetables are tender.

3. Ladle into serving bowls and sprinkle Parmesan cheese over the top of each if desired.

Nutritional Facts *(per serving)*: 250 calories, 15.5 g protein, 41.5 g carbohydrate, 3 g fat (1.3 g saturated fat, 1.1 g monounsaturated fat, 0.7 g polyunsaturated fat, 0.2 g omega-3 fatty acids, 0.5 g omega-6 fatty acids), 2 mg cholesterol, 8 g fiber, 679 mg sodium. Calories from fat: 12 percent.

890 RE vitamin A, 26 mg vitamin C, 1 IU vitamin D, 1.2 IU vitamin E, 0.3 mcg vitamin B$_{12}$, 108 mcg folate, 167 mg calcium, 10 mcg selenium.

Deluxe Spinach Salad
with Balsamic Dijon Dressing

Spinach is loaded with nutrients and fiber. Here is a flavorful salad featuring fresh spinach.

Makes 5 large servings • Serving size: 3 cups

2 cups Roma tomatoes, chopped

1 red or yellow bell pepper, seeded and
  finely chopped

1 15-ounce can red kidney beans, rinsed
  and drained

6 green onions, sliced or chopped

1 6-ounce jar artichoke hearts, packed
  in water

1 2¼ oz can sliced ripe black olives,
  drained (optional)

1 cup fresh basil leaves, washed and
  patted dry (tear large leaves in half)

10 cups fresh spinach leaves, washed and
  patted dry (tear large leaves in half)

3 tablespoons Parmesan cheese, grated

5 strips Louis Rich Less Fat Turkey
  Bacon, cooked over low heat until crisp,
  then crumbled

BALSAMIC DIJON DRESSING:

¼ cup balsamic vinegar

1 tablespoon honey

2 tablespoons fat-free sour cream

1½ teaspoons Dijon mustard

2 tablespoons olive oil

½ teaspoon ground pepper

1 large or 2 small garlic cloves, pressed or
  minced

1. In a large bowl, toss tomatoes, bell pepper, beans, onions, artichoke hearts, and olives if desired. Refrigerate until needed.

2. In small food processor, blender, or by whisking in a bowl, combine dressing ingredients and blend until smooth. Refrigerate until needed.

3. Right before serving, toss tomato-bean mixture with basil and spinach leaves. Drizzle with dressing (you may want to reserve a small amount of dressing for individual differences—guests can always add more). Sprinkle Parmesan cheese and bacon bits over the salad.

Nutritional Facts (*per serving*): 265 calories, 13 g protein, 34 g carbohydrate, 10 g fat (2.3 g saturated fat, 5.8 g monounsaturated fat, 1.6 g polyunsaturated fat, 0.3 g omega-3 fatty acids, 1.3 g omega-6 fatty acids), 15 mg cholesterol, 9 g fiber, 944 mg sodium. Calories from fat: 34 percent.

790 RE vitamin A, 121 mg vitamin C, 1 IU vitamin D, 4 IU vitamin E, 0.1 mcg vitamin B_{12}, 100 mcg folate, 193 mg calcium, 3 mcg selenium.

Macaroni and Broccoli Salad

This is a no frills for macaroni salad . . . but it is really easy to make and appeals to kids and discerning grown-ups alike. After adding the broccoli to this macaroni salad, you may never go back to plain macaroni salad. Trust me, it's a great addition!

Makes 6 servings • Serving size: 1⅓ cup

2 cups dry salad macaroni

3 cups broccoli florets, cut into
    bite-size pieces and lightly
    steamed or microwaved until
    just tender

3 green onions (white and part of green),
    finely chopped

2 teaspoons parsley flakes, or 2 tablespoons
    fresh parsley, finely chopped

¼ teaspoon salt

Freshly ground pepper to taste

2 tablespoons mayonnaise

¼ cup fat-free or light sour cream

3 eggs, hard-boiled and peeled

1. Cook the macaroni noodles, following directions on box (boil about 8 to 10 minutes). Drain noodles well, rinse with cold water, and let cool.

2. Place noodles in a serving bowl, along with broccoli, onions, parsley, salt, and pepper to taste. In a small bowl, blend mayonnaise with sour cream; add mayonnaise mixture to the noodles in serving bowl.

3. Peel the shells off the eggs and discard two of the cooked yolks. Chop remaining eggs (3 whites and 1 yolk) and stir into the macaroni mixture. Add more salt and pepper to taste, if desired. Let sit in the refrigerator overnight (if you've got time).

Nutritional Facts (*per serving*): 221 calories, 9 g protein, 30 g carbohydrate, 7 g fat (1.5 g saturated fat, 2.1 g monounsaturated fat, 2.7 g polyunsaturated fat, 0.1 g omega-3 fatty acids, 0.5 g omega-6 fatty acids), 110 mg cholesterol, 2 g fiber, 175 mg sodium. Calories from fat: 28 percent.

178 RE vitamin A, 34 mg vitamin C, 13 IU vitamin D, 1.4 IU vitamin E, 0.3 mcg vitamin B_{12}, 120 mcg folate, 55 mg calcium, 31 mcg selenium.

Easy Vegetable-Bean Salad

One serving of this salad will give you a dose of alpha and beta-carotene, folic acid, vitamin C, fiber, and plant-derived omega-3 fatty acids from the canola oil. If you want to make this more of a meal and you want to add omega-3 fatty acids from fish and some protein into the picture—you can stir in a can of albacore tuna. *Makes 8 servings • Serving size: ¾ cup*

3 cups carrots, diced or thinly sliced

3 cups broccoli florets, cut into bite-size pieces

1 15-ounce can kidney beans, rinsed and drained well

½ cup mild yellow or red onion, finely chopped (use less if desired)

½ cup less-fat bottled vinaigrette made with canola or olive oil (less-fat or light dressings have 4–6 grams of fat per serving)

1 6-ounce albacore tuna canned in water (optional)

1. Place carrot pieces in a microwave-safe covered dish with ¼ cup water and microwave on high about 3–5 minutes, or until just barely tender. Drain well and add to a medium-size serving bowl.

2. Place broccoli pieces in a microwave-safe covered dish with ¼ cup water and cook on high about 3–5 minutes, or until just barely tender. Drain well and add to the serving bowl.

3. Add beans, onion, vinaigrette, and tuna (if desired) to the serving bowl and toss well to blend.

Nutritional Facts *(per serving)*: 130 calories, 10 g protein, 17 g carbohydrate, 3 g fat (0.3 g saturated fat, 0.1 g monounsaturated fat, 0.3 g polyunsaturated fat, 0.2 g omega-3 fatty acids, 0.1 g omega-6 fatty acids), 6.5 mg cholesterol, 5 g fiber, 398 mg sodium. Calories from fat: 21 percent.

1572 RE vitamin A, 30 mg vitamin C, 34 IU vitamin D, 1.4 IU vitamin E, 0.1 mcg vitamin B_{12}, 55 mcg folate, 51 mg calcium, 19 mcg selenium.

Artichoke-Spinach Lasagna

If you are making this dish for some children or adults who may not like the feta cheese topping, just top half the lasagna with it so there is a choice for everyone!

Makes 8 servings • Serving size: 4½ x 1¾-inch piece

1 *onion, chopped*

1 *tablespoon garlic, minced or chopped*

1 *14.5-ounce can lower-sodium chicken or vegetable broth*

1 *tablespoon fresh rosemary, chopped*

1 *14-ounce can marinated artichoke hearts, drained and chopped*

1 *10-ounce box frozen chopped spinach, thawed and gently squeezed of excess water*

1 *28-ounce jar marinara sauce*

9 *Barilla No-Boil Lasagna Noodles*

3 *cups shredded part-skim mozzarella cheese*

GARLIC-HERB FETA TOPPING
(OPTIONAL):
Blend the following ingredients with a fork in small bowl:

5 *ounces reduced-fat feta cheese*

2 *teaspoons Italian seasoning*

½ *teaspoon garlic powder*

1. Preheat oven to 350 degrees. Coat a 9x13-inch baking dish with canola oil cooking spray.

2. Spray a large nonstick skillet with canola oil cooking spray and place over medium heat. Sauté onion and garlic for 3 minutes or until onion is just tender. Stir in broth and rosemary; bring to a boil. Stir in artichoke hearts and spinach; reduce heat to simmer, cover skillet, and cook for 5 minutes. Stir in marinara sauce.

3. Spread 1½ cups of the marinara mixture in the bottom of a prepared baking dish. Top with three of the noodles and ¾ cup of the mozzarella cheese. Repeat the layers two more times, ending with the marinara mixture and remaining mozzarella cheese. Sprinkle with the feta topping if desired.

4. Spray a large sheet of foil with canola oil cooking spray, then cover lasagna with the foil, coated-side-down. Bake for 40 minutes. Uncover and bake 15 minutes more, or until hot and bubbly. Let stand 10 minutes before cutting.

Nutritional Facts *(per serving)*: 299 calories, 20 g protein, 33 g carbohydrate, 10 g fat (5 g saturated fat, 2.6 g monounsaturated fat, 1.5 g polyunsaturated fat, 0.1 g omega-3 fatty acids, 0.2 g omega-6 fatty acids), 24 mg cholesterol, 6.3 g fiber, 840 mg sodium. Calories from fat: 30 percent.

424 RE vitamin A, 27 mg vitamin C, 0 IU vitamin D, 1 IU vitamin E, 0.4 mcg vitamin B_{12}, 91 mcg folate, 388 mg calcium, 1 mcg selenium.

Power Pesto Pasta

Makes 4 servings • Serving size: ¼ cup

1 cup fresh spinach leaves, stems removed, firmly packed

1 cup fresh basil leaves, firmly packed

⅓ cup Parmesan cheese, grated

¼ cup pine nuts (or walnuts), toasted (toast nuts in non-stick frypan or saucepan over medium-low heat, stirring frequently, until lightly browned) and chopped

¼ teaspoon salt (optional)

2 cloves garlic, minced or pressed (about 2 teaspoons)

2 tablespoons olive oil

¼ cup fat-free half-and-half

3–4 cups linguine, fettucine, or spaghetti noodles, cooked and drained

2 cups broccoli florets, steamed or microwaved till just tender

2 cups carrot slices, steamed or microwaved till just tender

1. Combine spinach and basil leaves, Parmesan, pine nuts, salt, garlic, olive oil, and half-and-half in food processor and pulse until pesto texture is formed. (This will be a lumpy paste.)
2. Add a tablespoon or two more of half-and-half if needed. Toss with noodles and vegetables. Reheat mixture in a large saucepan over low heat if needed.

Nutritional Facts *(per serving)*: 413 calories, 16.5 g protein, 56 g carbohydrate, 14.5 g fat (3 g saturated fat, 7.7 g monounsaturated fat, 3.1 g polyunsaturated fat, 0.3 g omega-3 fatty acids, 2.7 g omega-6 fatty acids), 6 mg cholesterol, 8 g fiber, 197 mg sodium. Calories from fat: 31 percent.

2213 RE vitamin A, 72 mg vitamin C, 15 IU vitamin D, 3.2 IU vitamin E, 0.1 mcg vitamin B_{12}, 184 mcg folate, 234 mg calcium, 34 mcg selenium.

Roasted Vegetable Fettuccine

Makes 3 servings • Serving size: 2½ cups

1 eggplant, trimmed and cut horizontally into ¼-inch-thick slices

1 red bell pepper, seeded and cut into 8 strips

1½ cups cauliflower florets, cut into bite-size pieces

⅓ cup julienned sun-dried tomato strips that have been rehydrated by microwaving in a small bowl with ⅓ cup water on high for 2 minutes, then drained

1 tablespoon olive oil

¼ cup lowfat milk or fat-free half-and-half

¼ cup Parmesan cheese, finely shredded

1 clove garlic, minced or pressed

3 cups cooked fettuccini noodles (about 6 ounces dried, uncooked)

1. Preheat broiler. Line a large baking sheet (or 2 small sheets) with foil. Spray the top of the foil generously with olive oil or canola oil cooking spray.

2. Place eggplant and red pepper strips on the foil. Spray the tops with cooking spray. Broil, watching carefully, until tops are lightly browned, about 5 minutes. Flip vegetables and broil until other sides are lightly browned, about 3 minutes.

3. Meanwhile, steam or cook cauliflower in the microwave until just tender, about 3 minutes, drain well, and set aside.

4. Place red pepper strips, sundried tomato, olive oil, milk or fat-free half-and-half, Parmesan cheese, and garlic in food processor. Process briefly until blended. Cut eggplant into strips. Toss with noodles, eggplant strips, and cauliflower florets.

Nutritional Facts (*per serving*): 350 calories, 14 g protein, 57 g carbohydrate, 8 g fat (2.3 g saturated fat, 4.4 g monounsaturated fat, 1.1 g polyunsaturated fat, 0.2 g omega-3 fatty acids, 0.9 g omega-6 fatty acids), 7 mg cholesterol, 8 g fiber, 282 mg sodium. Calories from fat: 21 percent.

346 RE vitamin A, 132 mg vitamin C, 10 IU vitamin D, 2 IU vitamin E, 0.1 mcg vitamin B$_{12}$, 163 mcg folate, 155 mg calcium, 33 mcg selenium.

Grilled Veggie Kabobs

There is something about grilled vegetables that really works. Even people who aren't crazy about vegetables seem to like them when they are grilled. You can use any combination of vegetables—just make sure you partially cook the veggies that will take a little longer to cook. This is a really simple recipe to get your started!

Makes about 8 servings • Serving size: 1 large kabob

2–3 cups broccoli florets

2 whole zucchini, cut into ½-inch thick coins

2 cups small mushrooms, rinsed and stems removed

1 red, orange, or yellow bell pepper, quartered and cut into large bite-size pieces

About 2–3 tablespoons lower-fat bottled garlic and herb or steak marinade

1. Start the coals if you are going to grill the kabobs.
2. Place broccoli in a microwave-safe dish. Add ¼ cup water, cover the dish, and microwave on high until halfway cooked, about 4 minutes.
3. Thread the various vegetables onto 8 long metal skewers, alternating vegetables. (For example, thread a zucchini coin, then a piece of bell pepper, then a broccoli floret, then a mushroom, and repeat one more time to complete the skewer.)

Note: To keep the vegetables from turning on the skewer while you are trying to turn them over and cook the other side, thread the vegetables onto 2 skewers for each kabob.

4. Brush the vegetables generously with the marinade.
5. Use a stovetop grill or grill about 6 inches from the coals for about 5 minutes per side.

Nutritional Facts (*per serving*): 37 calories, 3 g protein, 6 g carbohydrate, 1 g fat (0.1 g saturated fat, 0 g monounsaturated fat, 2.5 g polyunsaturated fat, 0.2 g omega-3 fatty acids, 0.5 g omega-6 fatty acids), 134 mg cholesterol, 3 g fiber, 99 mg sodium. Calories from fat: 28 percent.

388 RE vitamin A, 39 mg vitamin C, 0 IU vitamin D, 3.3 IU vitamin E, 3.7 mcg vitamin B_{12}, 192 mcg folate, 170 mg calcium, 38 mcg selenium.

Power Quesadilla

It might be a bit scary to add all these vegetables to your quesadilla—but it is surprisingly delicious, and you can't beat getting all these high-powered vegetables in this easy entrée!

Makes 1 large serving (or 2 small servings) • Serving size: large 8–9" quesadilla

2 white, whole-wheat, or high-fiber flour
    tortillas
⅓ cup reduced-fat Monterey Jack cheese,
    grated and packed
1 cup broccoli florets, finely chopped
2 fire-roasted green chiles (canned whole
    mild green chiles, e.g., Ortega)

2 green onions, chopped
1 tomato, sliced (discard ends)
Salsa of choice (such as mango-pineapple
    or other fruit blend, or more
    traditional salsa)

1. Heat a medium-size high-quality nonstick frying pan over medium-low heat. Coat pan with canola oil cooking spray and add 1 flour tortilla. Sprinkle grated cheese and broccoli evenly over the tortilla.
2. Split the chiles in two and lay the four chile strips evenly on top of the cheese. Sprinkle green onions over the top and lay tomato slices on top of them. Place remaining flour tortilla on top and spray the top with nonstick cooking spray.
3. When the bottom of the tortilla is lightly brown, carefully flip the quesadilla. When the bottom tortilla is lightly brown, transfer the quesadilla to a cutting board. Cut into wedges and serve with salsa.

Nutritional Facts *(per small serving—not including salsa with a flour tortilla)*: 320 calories, 14 g protein, 47 g carbohydrate, 9.4 g fat (4 g saturated fat, 2.8 g monounsaturated fat, 0.9 g polyunsaturated fat, 0.1 g omega-3 fatty acids, 8 g omega-6 fatty acids), 13 mg cholesterol, 5.2 g fiber, 539 mg sodium. Calories from fat: 26 percent.

203 RE vitamin A, 46 mg vitamin C, 0 IU vitamin D, 2.2 IU vitamin E, 0.2 mcg vitamin B_{12}, 129 mcg folate, 251 mg calcium, 18 mcg selenium.

Barley and Broccoli Bake

This recipe takes a while to bake in the oven, but it is so worth it. You might want to double the recipe if you have a family of four or more. This tastes great as a leftover the next day, too.

Makes 4 servings • Serving size: 1½ cups

1½ tablespoons canola oil

1 medium onion, chopped

1 cup uncooked pearl barley

⅓ cup pine nuts

3 green onions, thinly sliced

2 cups broccoli florets, coarsely chopped

1 cup fresh mushrooms (crimini if available), sliced

½ cup fresh parsley, chopped

¼ teaspoon salt (optional)

⅛ teaspoon pepper

2 14-ounce cans vegetable broth (chicken broth can be substituted)

1. Preheat oven to 350 degrees. Add canola oil to large ovenproof saucepan and heat over medium-high heat. Stir in the onion, barley, and pine nuts. Cook and stir until barley is lightly browned, about 3–4 minutes.

2. Mix in green onions, broccoli, mushrooms, parsley, salt if desired, pepper, and broth.

3. Bake, uncovered, for 1 hour and 15 minutes in oven or until liquid has been absorbed and barley is tender.

Nutritional Facts (*per serving*): 328 calories, 10 g protein, 51 g carbohydrate, 10.5 g fat (1.2 g saturated fat, 4.8 g monounsaturated fat, 3.8 g polyunsaturated fat, 0.6 g omega-3 fatty acids, 3 g omega-6 fatty acids), 0 mg cholesterol, 11 g fiber, 400 mg sodium. Calories from fat: 29 percent.

212 RE vitamin A, 42 mg vitamin C, 13 IU vitamin D, 3.3 IU vitamin E, 0 mcg vitamin B$_{12}$, 57 mcg folate, 64 mg calcium, 23 mcg selenium.

Herb-Roasted Winter Vegetables

I call this "herb-roasted" because of the fresh rosemary, dried oregano, and garlic used to flavor the sauce, which gets drizzled over the vegetables before they start baking. A serving contains 129 percent of the recommended daily intake for vitamin A and 75 percent for vitamin C!

Makes 6 servings • Serving size: about 2 cups

¾ pound new potatoes, quartered (if you are using medium-size red potatoes, cut into large, bite-size pieces)

¾ pound parsnips, quartered or cut into large bite-size pieces

1½ cups baby carrots

1 onion, cut into wedges then broken into large chunks

2 tablespoons olive oil

3 tablespoons lemon juice

1 tablespoon white wine or beer (any type of broth can be substituted)

1½ teaspoons garlic, minced or chopped

1 tablespoon fresh rosemary, chopped

1 tablespoon dried oregano

Salt and pepper to taste (optional)

½ eggplant, quartered and cut into ½-inch strips

1 red bell pepper, cut in half widthwise, seeded, then cut into ½-inch-wide strips

1. Preheat oven to 450 degrees. Coat a 13x9-inch baking dish with canola oil cooking spray. Combine potatoes, parsnips, carrots, and onion in a prepared baking dish.
2. Combine olive oil, lemon juice, wine, garlic, rosemary, oregano, and salt and pepper to taste (if desired) in a small food processor or electric mixer. Drizzle mixture over the vegetables and bake uncovered in the oven for 20 minutes.
3. Remove dish from oven and stir in eggplant and bell pepper strips. Toss well. Bake 15–20 minutes more or until the vegetables are tender and brown on the edges.

Nutritional Facts *(per serving)*: 146 calories, 3 g protein, 24 g carbohydrate, 5 g fat (0.7 g saturated fat, 3.7 g monounsaturated fat, 0.6 g polyunsaturated fat, 0.1 g omega-3 fatty acids, 0.5 g omega-6 fatty acids), 0 mg cholesterol, 7.5 g fiber, 23 mg sodium. Calories from fat: 30 percent.

1,059 RE vitamin A, 78 mg vitamin C, 0 IU vitamin D, 2.3 IU vitamin E, 0 mcg vitamin B$_{12}$, 71 mcg folate, 44 mg calcium, 2 mcg selenium.

Light Almond-Asparagus Rice Pilaf

We know we should switch to whole grains whenever possible, because they give us fiber, phytochemicals, and other vitamins and minerals that we don't get from refined grains. But while some us have no problem switching to brown rice and whole-grain bread, others find this difficult. For this recipe, you can use half brown and half basmati rice, if you prefer.

Makes 4 servings • Serving size: 1¼ cups

1 tablespoon canola oil

1 cup uncooked brown converted rice
  (Success brown rice can be used)

2¼ cups low-sodium chicken broth

¼ cup sliced or slivered almonds

¼ cup onion, diced

1 celery stalk, diced (about ⅓ cup)

2 cups asparagus spears, cut on a slight
  diagonal into 1-inch pieces

1 teaspoon dried parsley (or 1 tablespoon
  fresh parsley, finely chopped)

1. Add canola oil to a medium nonstick saucepan over medium heat. Add the brown rice and sauté until some of the rice turns light brown, about 3–5 minutes. As the rice is browning, microwave the chicken broth on high in an 8-cup glass measure (or similar) until broth begins to bubble, about 5–7 minutes.

2. When the rice has browned nicely, quickly add the hot broth to the saucepan with the rice. Cover the pan and reduce heat to low. Simmer for 30–40 minutes.

3. As the rice cooks, spray canola oil cooking spray in a medium nonstick skillet, and place over medium heat. Add almonds, onion, celery, parsley, and asparagus, and sauté until almonds are golden brown, about 3 minutes; set aside.

4. When rice has cooked for 20 minutes, remove it from the heat and stir in the almond-celery-onion mixture. Cover the saucepan and let sit for 5 minutes (or until the remaining liquid is absorbed and flavors have had time to blend. Serve!

Nutritional Facts (*per serving*): 203 calories, 7 g protein, 23 g carbohydrate, 9.5 g fat (1 g saturated fat, 4.8 g monounsaturated fat, 0.2 g polyunsaturated fat, 0.3 g omega-3 fatty acids, 1.7 g omega-6 fatty acids), 2 mg cholesterol, 3.5 g fiber, 77 mg sodium. Calories from fat: 42 percent.

36 RE vitamin A, 9 mg vitamin C, 0 IU vitamin D, 5.5 IU vitamin E, 0 mcg vitamin B_{12}, 85 mcg folate, 49 mg calcium, 1.5 mcg selenium.

Appendix

FOLIC ACID–RICH FOODS

FOOD	SERVING SIZE	AMOUNT OF FOLATE (mcg)	CALORIES
Brewer's yeast	2 TB	626	45
Spinach, fresh	2 cups chopped	218	25
Green soybeans	½ cup cooked	211	188
Lentils, cooked	½ cup	179	115
Romaine lettuce	2 cups fresh	152	18
Pinto beans, cooked	½ cup	147	117
Spinach, cooked	½ cup	130	21
Black beans, cooked	½ cup	128	114
Navy beans	½ cup	128	129
Kidney beans, cooked	½ cup	115	112
Black-eyed peas	½ cup	105	80
Broccoli, cooked	1 cup chopped	104	44
Pasta, white	1 cup	98	197
Soynuts (roasted soybeans)	½ cup	95	190
Asparagus spears	4	88	14
Flour tortilla	1 10-inch	88	115
Greens (collard and mustard)	½ cup cooked	51–88	17
Orange juice	1 cup fresh	75	112
Beets, cooked	½ cup cooked	68	37
Papaya	1 cup cubes	53	55
Vegetable or tomato juice	1 cup	51	56
Brussels sprouts	½ cup cooked	47	30
Crab, cooked	3.5 ounces	42	109
Tofu	½ cup raw	37	180

Source: ESHA Research Food Processor II Nutrition analysis and Nutrients in Food, Lippincott Williams & Wilkins, 2000.

Note: It is also not unusual to find foods such as cereals fortified with 100 percent of the U.S. RDA for folate.

Selenium-Rich Foods

FOOD	SERVING SIZE	SELENIUM (mcg)	CALORIES
Brazil nuts	¼ cup	1,035	230
Oysters, cooked	3.5 oz	115	72
White tuna (albacore), canned in water, drained	3.5 oz	65	135
Clams, steamed	3.5 oz	64	147
Sardines	3.5 oz	52	206
Pork tenderloin, cooked	3.5 oz	48	163
Crab, cooked	3.5 oz	40	109
Saltwater fish (all types)	3.5 oz	approx. 40	approx. 180
Whole-wheat pasta, cooked	1 cup	36	approx. 180
Pork chop, lean	3.5 oz cooked	35	202
Dark chicken meat (no skin)	3.5 oz cooked	30	208
White chicken meat (no skin)	3.5 oz cooked	30	164
Pasta, regular, cooked	1 cup	30	197
Lamb, lean cooked	3.5 oz	26	276
Sunflower seeds	¼ cup	26	186
Whole-wheat bread	2 slices	26	172
Bagel, plain	2.5 oz	23	187
Brown rice, cooked	1 cup	20	216
Oatmeal, cooked	1 cup	19	145
Flour tortilla	1 10-inch	17	115
Soynuts (roasted soybeans)	½ cup	17	190
Freshwater fish (all types)	3.5 oz	approx. 15	approx. 150
Egg	1 cooked	13	74
Cottage cheese, lowfat	½ cup	12	82
Tofu	½ cup	12	180
Pinto beans, cooked	½ cup	9	93
Yogurt, lowfat	1 cup	8	155

Source: *Nutrients in Food* by Elizabeth Hands, Lippincott Williams & Wilkins Publishing, 2000, plus data from ESHA Research Food Processor II nutritional analysis software.

Beta-Carotene-Rich Fruits and Vegetables

Which specific fruits and vegetables reign as top food sources of each? Check out the top twenty list below. (Notice that quite a few of the fruits and vegetables are in both lists.)

Apricots

Artichoke hearts

Broccoli

Butternut squash

Cantaloupe

Carrots

Greens (beet, collard, and mustard)

Kale

Mango

Prunes

Pumpkin

Red peppers

Romaine and green leaf lettuce

Spinach

Sweet potato

Swiss chard

Tomato juice and tomato sauce

Vitamin C–Rich Fruits and Vegetables

Blackberries

Broccoli

Brussels sprouts

Butternut squash

Cantaloupe

Cauliflower

Grapes

Green pepper

Greens (collard, beet, and mustard)

Green soybeans

Kale

Kiwifruit

Mango

Orange and grapefruit juice (fresh)

Oranges

Papaya

Pink/red/white grapefruit

Potato

Raspberries

Red cabbage

Red peppers

Snap peas

Strawberries

Swiss chard

Tomatoes and tomato sauce

Tomato-vegetable or tomato juice

B_{12}-RICH FOODS

FOOD	SERVING SIZE	AMOUNT OF B_{12} (mcg)	CALORIES
Clams	3.5 oz steamed	99	147
Oysters	3.5 oz cooked	27	136
Herring	3.5 oz cooked	10	248
Crab	3.5 oz cooked	9	101
Trout	3.5 oz cooked	6	149
Pollock (fish)	3.5 oz cooked	4	112
Catfish	3.5 oz cooked	3	168
Salmon	3.5 oz cooked	3	180
Light tuna, canned in water	3.5 oz canned	3	115
Beef (lean)	3.5 oz cooked	2.5	174
Lamb (lean)	3.5 oz cooked	2.7	202
Shrimp	3.5 oz cooked	1.5	98
Lowfat yogurt	1 cup	1.4	155
Nonfat milk	1 cup	0.93	85
Whole milk	1 cup	0.9	150
Cottage cheese lowfat 1%	½ cup	0.8	82
Pork (lean)	3.5 oz cooked	0.6	163
Egg	1 cooked	0.5	75
Swiss or provolone cheese	1 oz	0.5	107
Turkey (light or dark meat)	3.5 oz cooked	0.4	186
Chicken, light meat skinless, roasted	3.5 oz cooked	0.4	164
Chicken, dark meat skinless, roasted	3.5 oz cooked	0.3	208

Note: Organ meats, including various livers and kidneys, are high in B_{12} but are not included in the list due to their high amount of cholesterol, saturated fat, and potential toxins.

MAGNESIUM-RICH FOODS

FOOD	SERVING SIZE	MAGNESIUM (mg)	CALORIES
Almonds	¼ cup	120	212
Artichokes	1 whole	72	60
Beet greens, cooked	½ cup	49	20
Black beans, cooked	½ cup	60	114
Black-eyed peas, cooked	½ cup	43	80
Brazil nuts	¼ cup	83	230
Brown rice, cooked	½ cup	42	108
Cashews	¼ cup	79	196
Filberts	¼ cup	96	213
Fish (average), cooked, such as salmon and halibut	3.5 ounces	40–106 (approximately)	139–180
Flaxseeds, ground	2 tablespoons	80	around 60
Kidney beans, cooked	½ cup	40	109
King crab, cooked	3.5 ounces	43	137
Lowfat yogurt	1 cup	43	155
Blackstrap molasses	1 tablespoon	50	48
Navy beans/baked beans/ baby limas	½ cup	52	129
Oatmeal, cooked	1 cup	56	145
Okra, cooked	½ cup	46	25
Peanuts	¼ cup	63	214
Peanut butter	2 tablespoons	57	191
Pistachios	¼ cup	50	183
Pumpkin seeds, roasted	¼ cup	42	71
Soynuts, roasted	¼ cup	98	200
Spinach, cooked	½ cup	66	21
Sunflower seeds	¼ cup	127	205
Swiss chard, cooked	½ cup	75	18
Firm tofu	¼ cup	60	90
Walnuts	¼ cup	50	160

MAGNESIUM-RICH FOODS *(continued)*

FOOD	SERVING SIZE	MAGNESIUM (mg)	CALORIES
Wheat germ	2 tablespoons	45	54
Whole-wheat pasta, cooked	1 cup	42	174

Source: *Nutrients in Food,* 2000, Lippincott Williams & Wilkins)

CALCIUM-RICH DAIRY FOODS

FOOD	SERVING SIZE	CALCIUM (mgs) (APPROXIMATE VALUES)	CALORIES
American cheese	1 ounce	174	106
Cheese (regular and reduced-fat)	1 ounce	185	106
Cottage cheese, lowfat	½ cup	70	82
Evaporated skim milk	¼ cup	185	50
Fat-free sour cream	½ cup	142	124
Instant hot cocoa	1 packet	100 (check labels because the brands vary)	103
Lowfat frozen yogurt	½ cup	105	around 114
Milk, nonfat or 1 percent lowfat	1 cup	300	around 102
Milk, whole or buttermilk	1 cup	280	around 150
Nonfat dry milk powder	1 ounce	350	101
Parmesan cheese	1 ounce shredded	350	118
Ricotta cheese, part-skim	¼ cup	165	85
Vanilla ice milk or light ice cream	½ cup	109	92
Yogurt, lowfat flavored	1 cup	300	250
Yogurt, nonfat or lowfat plain	1 cup	400	155

Calcium-Rich Plant and Fish foods

FOOD	SERVING SIZE	CALCIUM (mgs)	CALORIES
Acorn squash, cooked	1 cup	90	115
Almonds	¼ cup	92	212
Bass, trout, or halibut, baked	3 ounces	75	about 120
Beans (navy, pinto, or kidney), cooked	½ cup	50	109
Black-eyed peas, cooked	½ cup	100	80
Blackstrap molasses	1 tablespoon	175	48
Broccoli, cooked	1 cup	75	44
Bok choy, cooked	½ cup	79	10
Butternut squash, cooked	1 cup	84	82
Clams, steamed/boiled/canned	3 ounces	80	126
Crab, cooked	3 ounces	89	87
Filberts and Brazil nuts	¼ cup	64	213
Greens (collard, turnip, beet, etc.), cooked	½ cup	80–100	14
Instant plain oatmeal	1 packet	150	104
Kale, cooked	½ cup	50	21
Loose-leaf lettuce	2 cups	76	20
Ocean perch, baked	3 ounces	120	107
Okra, cooked	1 cup	100	51
Orange segments	1 cup	72	85
Salmon, canned	3 ounces	200	120
Sardines canned in water	3.5 ounces	84	215
Shrimp, cooked	3 ounces	35	84
Soybeans, green, cooked	½ cup	252	188
Soymilk, fresh (some brands)	1 cup	240	80
Soynuts, roasted soybeans	½ cup	119	400
Spinach, raw	2 cups	111	25
Spinach, cooked	½ cup	140	21
Swiss chard, cooked	½ cup	51	18
Tofu, firm	½ cup	200–250	181

Resources

CHAPTER ONE: WHY LIVE HRT-FREE?

Beral, V., et al. "Breast Cancer and Hormone Replacement Therapy in the Million Woman Study." *Lancet* 362:419–27, 2003.

Cauley, Jane A., et al. "Effects of Hormone Replacement Therapy on Clinical Fractures and Height Loss: The Heart and Estrogen/Progestin Replacement Study." *American Journal of Medicine* 110:442–50, 2001.

Clemons, M., and P. Goss. "Mechanisms of Disease: Estrogen and the Risk of Breast Cancer." *New England Journal of Medicine* 344:276–85, 2001.

Collaborative Group on Hormonal Factors in Breast Cancer. "Breast Cancer and Hormone Replacement Therapy: Collaborative Re-analysis of Data from 51 Epidemiological Studies of 52, 705 Women with Breast Cancer and 108, 411 Women without Breast Cancer." *Lancet* 350:1047–59, 1997.

Cummings, Steven R., M.D., et al. "Effect of Alendronate on Risk of Fracture in Women with Low Bone Density but Without Vertebral Fractures." *Journal of the American Medical Association* 280:2077–82, 1998.

Fuchs-Young, R., et al. "Raloxifene is a Tissue-Sensitive Agonist/Antagonist That Functions Through the Estrogen Receptor." *Annals of the New York Academy of Sciences* 761:355–60, 1995.

Grady, Deborah, et al. "Postmenopausal Hormone Therapy Increases Risk of Venous Thromboembolic Disease." *Annals of Internal Medicine* 132:689–96, 2000.

Greendale, G. A., et al. "Symptom Relief and Side Effects of Postmenopausal Hormones: Results from the Postmenopausal Estrogen/Progestin Interventions Trial." *Obstetrics and Gynecology* 92:982–88, 1998.

Herrington, D. M., et al. "Effects of Estrogen Replacement on the Progression of Coronary-Artery Atherosclerosis." *New England Journal of Medicine* 343:522–29, 2000.

Hulley, S., et al. "Randomized Trial of Estrogen Plus Progestin for Secondary Prevention of Coronary Heart Disease in Postmenopausal Women." *Journal of the American Medical Association,* 280:605–13, 1998.

MacLennan, A. H., S. Lester, and V. Moore. "Oral Estrogen Replacement Therapy Versus Placebo for Hot Flushes: A Systematic Review." *Climacteric* 4 (1): 58–74, 2001.

Mosca, Lori, et al. "Hormone Replacement Therapy and Cardiovascular Disease: A Statement for Healthcare Professionals from the American Heart Association." *Circulation* 104:499–503, 2001.

National Heart, Lung, and Blood Institute. "Women's Health Initiative Hormone Replacement Study Fact Sheets." www.nhlbi.nih.gov, 2002.

———. Communications Office. "Preliminary Trends in Women's Health Initiative." 2000.

Simon, Joel A., et al. "Effect of Estrogen Plus Progestin on Risk for Biliary Tract Surgery in Postmenopausal Women with Coronary Artery Disease." *Annals of Internal Medicine* 135:493–501, 2001.

Torgerson, David J., Ph.D., and S. Bell-Syer, M.Sc. "Hormone Replacement Therapy and Prevention of Nonvertebral Fractures: A Meta-analysis of Randomized Trials." *Journal of the American Medical Association* 285:2891–97, 2001.

Viscoli, C. M., et al. "A Clinical Trial of Estrogen-Replacement Therapy After Ischemic Stroke." *New England Journal of Medicine* 345:1243–49, 2001.

Writing Group for the Postmenopausal Estrogen/Progestin Intervention trial. "Effects of Hormone Replacement Therapy on Bone Mineral Density: Results from the Postmenopausal Estrogen/ Progestin Intervention (PEPI) Trial." *Journal of the American Medical Association* 276:1389–96, 1996.

Writing Group for the Women's Health Initiative. "Risk and Benefits of Estrogen Plus Progestin in Healthy Postmenopausal Women: Principal Results from the Women's Health Initiative Randomized Controlled Trial." *Journal of the American Medical Association* 228:321–53, 2002.

CHAPTER TWO: IS IT ME, OR IS IT HOT IN HERE?

Yamamoto, Seiichiro. "Soy, Isoflavones, and Breast Cancer Risk in Japan." *Journal of the National Cancer Institute* 95 (12):906–13.

CHAPTER FIVE: APHRODISIACS FOR MENOPAUSAL WOMEN ONLY

Murphy, L. L., et al. "Ginseng, Sex Behavior, and Nitric Oxide." *Annals of the New York Academy of Sciences* 962:372–77, 2002.

Murray, W. "Decreased Libido in Postmenopausal Women." *Nurse Practitioner's Forum* 11 (4): 219–24, 2000.

Nocerino, E., et al. "The Aphrodisiac and Adaptogenic Properties of Ginseng." *Fitoterapia* 71 (Suppl 1): S1–5, 2000.

CHAPTER SIX: I'M NOT MOODY—I'M THIS CRANKY ALL THE TIME!

Benton, David. "Selenium Intake, Mood, and Other Aspects of Psychological Functioning." *Nutritional Neuroscience* 5 (6): 363–74, 2002.

Heinz, Andreas, et al. "Serotonergic Dysfunction, Negative Mood States, and Response to Alcohol." *Alcohol Clinical and Experimental Research* 25 (4): 487–95, 2001.

"Identifying and Promoting the Specific Nutrition and Physical Activity Needs of Women Aged 40 and Over." *Medical Journal of Australia* 173:S104–5, 2000.

Markus, C. R., et al. "Does Carbohydrate-rich, Protein-poor Food Prevent a Deterioration of Mood and Cognitive Performance of Stress-Prone Subjects When Subjected to a Stressful Task?" *Appetite* 31 (1): 49–65, 1998.

Mayo Clinic. "Your Mind: Experiencing the Emotion and Cognitive Changes of Midlife." *Women's Health Source* December 2002, p. 4.

CHAPTER SEVEN: WHAT WAS I SAYING? I MUST BE HAVING ONE OF THOSE MENOPAUSE MOMENTS

Deijer, J. B., et al. "Tyrosine Improves Cognitive Performance and Reduces Blood Pressure in Cadets After One Week of a Combat Training Course." *Brain Research Bulletin* 48 (2): 203–9, 1999.

Ling, J., et al. "Effects of Alcohol on Subjective Ratings of Everyday Memory Deficits." Alcoholism: *Clinical and Experimental Research* 27 (6): 970–4, 2003.

Solomon, Paul R. "Gingko for Memory Enhancement: A Randomized Controlled Trial." *Journal of the American Medical Association* 288:835–40, 2002.

Wurtman, R. J., and J. J. Wurtman. "Brain Serotonin, carbohydrate-craving, obesity and depression." *Obesity Research* 3 (Suppl 4): 477S–80S, 1995.

CHAPTER EIGHT: IF I'M SWEATING SO MUCH, WHY AREN'T I LOSING WEIGHT?

Bhathena, Sam J., and Manuel T. Velasquez. "Beneficial Role of Dietary Phytoestrogens in Obesity and Diabetes." *American Journal of Clinical Nutrition* 76:1191–201, 2002.

Davies, M. K. "Calcium Intake and Body Weight." *Journal of Clinical Endocrinology* 85:4635, 2000.

Jacquain, M., et al. "Calcium Intake and Body Composition in Adults." *Obesity Research* 175S:PF104, 2001.

Ogden, J. "The Correlates of Long-Term Weight Loss: A Group Comparison Study of Obesity." *International Journal of Obesity* 24:1018–25, 2000.

Pitsavos, Christos. "The Adoption of Mediterranean Diet Attenuates the Development of Acute Coronary Syndrome in People with Metabolic Syndrome." *Nutrition* Mar 19 (3): 253–56, 2003.

Sarlio-Lahteenkorva, S., A. Rissanen, and J. Kaprio. "A Descriptive Study of Weight-Loss Maintenance: 6- and 15-year Follow-up of Initially Overweight Adults." *International Journal of Obesity* 24 (1):116–25, 2000.

Weigle, David S., et al. "Roles of Leptin and Ghrelin in the Loss of Body Weight Caused by Low Fat, High Carbohydrate Diet." *Journal of Clinical Endocrinology & Metabolism* 88:1577–86, 2003.

Zemel, M. B. "Calcium Modulation of Hypertension and Obesity: Mechanisms and Implications." *Journal of the American College of Nutrition* 20:428S–35S, 2001.

Zemel, M. B., et al. "Dietary Calcium and Dairy Products Accelerate Weight and Fat Loss During Energy Restriction in Obese Adults." *American Journal of Clinical Nutrition* 75:342S, 2002.

Zemel, M. B., et al. "Regulation of Adiposity by Dietary Calcium." *Federation of American Societies for Experimental Biology Journal* 14:1132, 2000.

CHAPTER NINE: BOOST YOUR BONES NATURALLY

Board of Trustees of the North American Menopause Society. "Management of Postmenopausal Osteoporosis: Position Statement of the North American Menopause Society." *Menopause* 9 (2): 84–101, 2002.

Davidson, Michelle, CNM, Ph.D. "Pharmacotherapeutics for Osteoporosis Prevention and Treatment." *Journal of Midwifery & Women's Health* 48:39, 2003.

Feskanich, Diane, et al. "Walking and Leisure-Time Activity and Risk of Hip Fracture in Post-menopausal Women." *Journal of the American Medical Association* 288:2300–06, 2002.

Reid, Ian R., M.D. "Therapy of Osteoporosis: Calcium, Vitamin D, and Exercise." *American Journal of Medical Sciences* 312 (6): 278–86, 1996.

Ricci, Trina A., et al. "Calcium Supplementation Suppresses Bone Turnover During Weight Reduction in Postmenopausal Women." *Journal of Bone Mineral Research* 13 (6): 1045–50, 1998.

CHAPTER TEN: HOW TO REDUCE YOUR RISK OF COLON CANCER WITHOUT HRT

American Dietetic Association. "Position of the ADA: Health Implications of Dietary Fiber." *Journal of the American Dietetic Association* 102 (7): 993–1000, 2002.

American Institute for Cancer Research Newsletter. "A Closer Look at Colon Cancer." Spring 2003.

Calle, E. E., et al. "Overweight, Obesity, and Mortality from Cancer in a Prospectively Studied Cohort of U.S. Adults." *New England Journal of Medicine* 348:1625–38, 2003.

Dragsted, Lars O., et al. "A Sucrose-rich Diet Induces Mutations in the Rat Colon." *Cancer Research* 62 (15): 4339–45, 2002.

Fuchs, Charles S., et al. "The Influence of Folate and Multivitamin Use on the Familial Risk of Colon Cancer in Women." *Cancer Epidemiology Biomarkers & Prevention* 11:227–34, 2002.

Kato, Taeko, et al. "Influence of Omega-3 Fatty Acids on the Growth of Human Colon Carcinoma in Nude Mice." *Cancer Letters* 187 (1–2): 169–77, 2002.

Kim, Daniel J. "Report from a Symposium on Diet and Breast Cancer." *Cancer Causes and Control* 13:591–94, 2002.

Konings, Erik J. M., et al. "Intake of Dietary Folate and Vitamins and Risk of Colorectal Carcinoma: Results from the Netherlands Cohort Study." *Cancer* 95 (7): 1421–33, 2002.

Kris-Etherton, Penny M., et al. "Bioactive Compounds in Foods: Their Role in the Prevention of Cardiovascular Disease and Cancer." *American Journal of Medicine* 113 (Suppl 9.2): 71–88, 2002.

Matos, Elena, and Aldo Brandani. "Review on Meat Consumption and Cancer in South America." *Mutation Research* 506–7:243–49, 2002.

Rock, Cheryl L., and Wendy Demark-Wahnefried. "Can Lifestyle Modification Increase Survival in Women Diagnosed with Breast Cancer?" *Journal of Nutrition* 132 (Suppl 11): 3504S–7S, 2002.

Index